Dear Reader:

Vitamins are very important in the overall health and well-being of your child. Vitamin C plays a key role in contributing to the child's health development. Specifically, Vitamin C is essential in the formation of bone, cartilage, and connective tissue, and important for the growth and repair of a child's tissue cells, gums, blood vessels, bones, and teeth.

Apple Juice is one of the first foods that pediatricians recommend for babies, and kids enjoy it all through their lives.

I am very pleased that Seneca Foods Corporation has selected "Vitamin Bible For Your Kids" to participate in their "A, B, Vitamin C" Sweepstakes Program. Seneca has long recognized the importance of Vitamin C in your child's diet, and has made a special effort to ensure that each glass of Seneca Apple Juice has a full day's supply of Vitamin C. In fact, Seneca is the only apple juice enriched with Vitamin C.

I hope you will enjoy the benefits of the "Vitamin Bible For Your Kids" and Seneca Apple Juice for years to come.

Dr. Earl Mindell

Earl Mindell's VITAMIN BIBLE FOR YOUR KIDS

EARL L. MINDELL, R.Ph., Ph.D

BANTAM BOOKS
TORONTO • NEW YORK • LONDON • SYDNEY

This book is dedicated to
my wonderful children.

ALANNA and EVAN,

my wife, GAIL,

our parents and families,
and to the health and happiness
of children everywhere.

*This low-priced Bantam Book
has been completely reset in a type face
designed for easy reading, and was printed
from new plates. It contains the complete
text of the original hard-cover edition.*
NOT ONE WORD HAS BEEN OMITTED.

EARL MINDELL'S VITAMIN BIBLE FOR YOUR KIDS

*A Bantam Book / published by arrangement with
Rawson, Wade Publishers Inc.*

PRINTING HISTORY
*Rawson, Wade edition published October 1981
A Selection of Rodale Press Book Club January 1982
Bantam edition / November 1982*

ISBN 0-553-22660-6

Published simultaneously in the United States and Canada

---

*Bantam Books are published by Bantam Books, Inc. Its trademark,
consisting of the words "Bantam Books" and the portrayal of a
rooster, is Registered in U.S. Patent and Trademark Office and in
other countries. Marca Registrada. Bantam Books, Inc., 666 Fifth
Avenue, New York, New York 10103.*

PRINTED IN THE UNITED STATES OF AMERICA

O   0 9 8 7 6 5 4

ACKNOWLEDGMENTS

I wish to express my deep and lasting appreciation to my many friends and associates who have assisted me in the preparation of this book, especially J. Kenny, Ph.D., Linus Pauling, Ph.D., Robert Mendelson, M.D., Arnold Fox, M.D., Gershon Lesser, M.D., David Velkoff, M.D., Bernard Bubman, R.Ph., Mel Rich, R. Ph., and Hester Mundis.

I would also like to thank the International College of Applied Nutrition, the Nutrition Foundation, the International Academy of Preventative Medicine, the American Academy of Pediatrics, the American Dietetic Association, the American Pharmaceutical Association, the National Dairy Council, the National Academy of Sciences, the Society for Nutrition Education, the United Fresh Fruit and Vegetable Association, the U.S. Department of Health, Education and Welfare, Health Services Administration; Betty Haskins, Peter Mallory, Judy Beal, Susan Schwartz, and Richard Curtis, whose resources and encouragement were integral to the success of my project.

Contents

1. Why your kids need vitamins 2. What vitamins really are 3. How they work for your kids 4. Take care of your baby *before* it's born 5. Increased needs during pregnancy 6. What mothers-to-be should know about drugs 7. Any questions about chapter I?

8. Let's start with vitamin A 9. Vitamin B_1 (Thiamine) 10. Vitamin B_2 (Riboflavin) 11. Vitamin B_6 (Pyridoxine) 12. Vitamin B_{12} (Cobalamin) 13. Vitamin B_{13} (Orotic Acid) 14. B_{15} (Pangamic Acid) 15. Vitamin B_{17} (Laetrile) 16. Biotin (Coenzyme R or Vitamin H) 17. Vitamin C (Ascorbic Acid, Cevitamic Acid) 18. Calcium Pantothenate (Pantothenic Acid, Panthenol, Vitamin B_5) 19. Choline 20. Vitamin D (Calciferol, Viosterol, Ergosterol, "Sunshine Vitamin") 21. Vitamin E (Tocopherol) 22. Vitamin F (Unsaturated Fatty Acids—Linoleic, Linolenic, and Arachidonic) 23. Folic Acid (Folacin) 24. Inositol 25. Vitamin K (Menadione) 26. Niacin (Nicotinic Acid, Niacinamide, Nicotinamide) 27. Vitamin P (C Complex, Citrus Bioflavonoids, Rutin, Hesperidin) 28. PABA (Para-aminobenzoic Acid) 29. Vitamin T 30. Vitamin U 31. Any questions about chapter II?

32. Calcium 33. Chlorine 34. Chromium 35. Cobalt 36. Copper 37. Fluorine 38. Iodine (Iodide) 39. Iron 40. Magnesium 41. Manganese 42. Molybdenum 43. Phosphorus 44. Potassium 45. Selenium 46. Sodium

47. Sulfur 48. Vanadium 49. Zinc 50. Any questions about chapter III?

51. Water 52. Protein—the Superstar Nutrient 53. Facts and fallacies about protein 54. How much does my child really need? 55. How to sneak more into your child's diet 56. Caring about carbohydrates 57. The importance of fats 58. Knowing the fats 59. Calorie requirements from infancy to adolescence 60. Yea, for Yeast! 61. Any questions about chapter IV?

62. Why parents must be detectives 63. Causes of vitamin deficiencies in children 64. Deficiency diseases, symptoms, and warning signals 65. Tests for deficiencies 66. Hypervitaminosis—how to spot it 67. Hypervitaminosis—how to avoid it 68. How and when to administer vitamins to children 69. What to look for when buying vitamins for children 70. Any questions about chapter V?

71. Be cautious when you mix kids and vitamins 72. Any questions about chapter VI?

73. The pros and cons 74. You have to be twice as careful when you're feeding two 75. Some facts about formulas 76. Special formulas for special situations 77. Any questions about chapter VII?

78. Milk facts that moms (and dads) should know 79. How much milk do kids *really* need? 80. How do substitutes stack up? 81. Delicious treats that even

milk-haters love 82. Yogurt is more than yummy 83. Any questions about chapter VIII?

84. Starting solid foods 85. Solid facts 86. Catering to baby's invisible sweet tooth 87. Baby's food allergies 88. Making your own baby food is easier than you thought 89. Any questions about chapter IX?

90. What are balanced meals? 91. The four food groups— and what your child needs from each 92. How big is a serving? 93. Why breakfast is important 94. What's in those cereal boxes? 95. Making the best of a bad situation 96. Not-so-sweet mysteries about cereals revealed 97. How to convert nonbreakfast-eaters 98. School lunches 99. Some of the best lunches come in brown bags 100. Why your child doesn't have to eat spinach or liver 101. Any questions about chapter X?

102. What your kids are eating at those fast-food places 103. The junk food connection 104. How sweet it isn't 105. A matter of Hide-and-Sweet 106. Watch out! Caffeine is not just in coffee 107. How to help your child break the junk-food habit 108. Snacking can be healthy 109. Any questions about chapter XI?

110. What an allergy is 111. Types of food allergies 112. Possible symptoms of hidden food allergies 113. Preventing allergies 114. Tests for allergies 115. Milk-free diets 116. Egg-free diets 117. Wheat-free diets 118. Corn-

A NOTE TO PARENTS

The regimens throughout this book are recommendations, not prescriptions, and are not intended as medical advice. Before starting your child on any new program, you should check with a nutritionally oriented doctor, especially if the child has any physical problems or conditions or is taking any medication.

Preface

In my many talks during the past few years with concerned mothers and fathers across the country, I discovered that confusion and misinformation abound in one area above all others—that of children's nutrition. Because of this, I realized that what parents and parents-to-be needed was a nutritional self-defense manual—a simplified guide that not only would tell them all they wanted to know about how vitamins and nutrients really influenced their child's physical and emotional development but also would offer them practical solutions to particular problems. The result is this book.

Speaking plainly as a pharmacist, a nutritionist, and a parent, I have attempted to provide answers for those of you who want the best nutrition for your child but don't know how to go about it; those of you who think it's impossible to get your child to eat natural foods while his peers are still munching Twinkies and Ding-Dongs; those of you who want to keep your kids well without constantly resorting to prescription medicines; those of you who want to know exactly how to tell when vitamins are called for and when they're not, what foods supply them and what medicines deplete them, how much is enough and how much is too much.

Because I am convinced that there are no bad children, only bad diets, and that good nutrition should begin as early as possible—even before the child is born—I've included advice for pregnant women and for nursing mothers. And because I also feel that children should not be statistics, that every child is special in his or her own way, I have tried to individualize information so that you can more easily relate it to *your* child.

In my effort to simplify this vast amount of information, I've used the word *he* throughout the book in its generic sense, but I fully intend it to mean both *he* and *she*. (My wife and daughter have forgiven me, so I hope you will, too.)

I'm well aware that parents often have no time to read the newspaper, let alone a book from cover to cover, and for this reason I've arranged this guide in numbered quick-reference sections so that you can find answers to particular questions about your child at a glance. Although I've tried to make all my recommendations for diets and supplements as specific as possible, none of them are meant to be prescriptive and they should not be taken as medical advice. Rather, they are to be used as a guide in working with your child's physician. Bear in mind, too, that when brand names appear, they are strictly for informational purposes.

With statistics showing that children actually eat more cake, cookies, and doughnuts than meat and more candy than eggs and that they drink more soda than milk, I feel that the time for preventive nutrition has come. Parents have to fight back against the onslaught of processed and refined (essentially junk) foods that are robbing our kids of their right to optimum health and the full realization of their natural potential. My fondest hope is that this book will provide you and your children with the nutritional ammunition necessary to win the battle and reap the rewards for years to come.

EARL L. MINDELL, R. Ph., Ph.D.

Part One

THE
BASICS

CHAPTER I

Why Vitamins Are
as Important as Love

1. Why your kids need vitamins

Vitamins are essential to your child's physical, emotional, and mental growth; indeed, they are as important as love. The only difference, perhaps, is that you can never oversupply love. During the first year of life, a child usually triples his birth weight. This phenomenal rate of growth is made possible only by sufficient calories and adequate nutrients. The calories are provided by the metabolism of fats, proteins, and carbohydrates, but without essential vitamins and minerals, proper metabolism could not take place. In effect, a proper vitamin level is essential to healthy children and the foundation for healthy adults.

> *An infant does not naturally get adequate vitamins during the first year of life.*

What children eat determines not only how much they weigh but also how well they feel and perform (and, of course, how they look). Because a child's growing brain has at least double the energy requirements of an adult's—and because it is incapable of storing the glucose energy it needs—it must constantly be provided with food. But calories alone are not enough, which is why almost all infants—breast- or bottle-fed—are given supplementary vitamins. A newborn child does not normally have an adequate vitamin intake during the first year of life, since neither cow's milk nor breast milk is an ample source. For this reason, and because it is difficult to tell how well food is being absorbed from the intestinal tract, the general rule is to provide infants and children with extra vitamins to make sure that no possible deficiency develops at this important formative stage.

2. What vitamins really are

Vitamins are nutrients—organic substances necessary for life. They are essential to the normal functioning of our bodies and, with a few exceptions, cannot be manufactured or synthesized internally. Along with other nutrients, such as minerals, proteins, fats, carbohydrates, and water, they make it possible for children to move, think, learn and grow. In their natural state, vitamins are found in minute quantities in all food. They must be obtained from these foods or from dietary supplements, which are available in tablet, capsule, liquid, or injection forms.

- Each vitamin does its own unique work.
- No vitamin can substitute for another or do the work of any other nutrient.
- About fifty nutrients are needed to build, maintain, and regulate body processes.
- It is impossible to sustain life without all the essential vitamins.

> *Vitamins must be obtained from foods or dietary supplements in order to sustain life.*

3. How they work for your kids

Vitamins are components of the enzyme systems, which, in a sense, power your child. Enzyme systems act like spark plugs: they energize and regulate your child's metabolism and keep him tuned up and functioning at peak performance.

Minute as these food substances are, a single deficiency can endanger the whole body. (A lack of vitamin A alone, for example, can cause a marked loss of vision, mental and physical retardation, anemia, kidney infection, bronchial tube inflammation, and poor tooth formation.) On the other hand, too much of a good thing, even vitamin A, can cause problems, too. (See section 66, Hypervitaminosis.)

4. Take care of your baby before it's born

Since healthy mothers have healthier babies, the best thing a pregnant woman can do for her unborn infant is to make certain that the child is being supplied with sufficient nutrients.

> *The old belief that the baby takes what he needs from the mother's body no matter what she eats is untrue.*

A pregnant woman must provide a constant supply of good nutrients for the proper building of the child's body tissues. A baby will take what he needs from the mother's body, often dangerously depleting her of calcium and other minerals and vitamins. This can result in a difficult labor or premature birth or can even affect her ability to nurse, but the baby can take only what's *there*. If a mother-to-be is deficient in nutrients, the child will suffer for it, too.

Mounting evidence, including an extensive study done recently by Professor Derek Bryce-Smith in Britain, shows that behavioral disorders and impaired development *can* be linked to diet factors during fetal life.

The major stages in the embryo's development occur during the first few weeks of life, before most women even know that they're pregnant. Because of this, it's wise for women contemplating motherhood to consider the advantages of shaping up nutritionally *before* conception.

BE SURE YOUR DIET INCLUDES:

Foods that contain B-complex vitamins (nutritional yeast, liver, leafy green vegetables, cheese, fish eggs)

Foods that contain folic acid (carrots, cantaloupe, beans, whole wheat and dark rye flour)

Foods that contain vitamin C (citrus fruits, strawberries, tomatoes, cauliflower, green and leafy vegetables)

Foods that contain calcium (milk, milk products, cheese, soybeans, peanuts, walnuts, dried beans, green vegetables)

TO GET THE MOST VITAMINS FROM THESE FOODS:

- Wash but don't soak fresh vegetables (you'll lose vitamins B and C).
- Cut fruits and vegetables when you're ready to eat them. (They lose vitamins when left standing.)
- Cook vegetables quickly in smallest amount of water.
- Don't thaw frozen vegetables before cooking.
- Use converted and parboiled rice instead of polished rice. (Brown rice is more nutritious than white.)
- Know that iron cooking pots can give you the benefit of that mineral but can shortchange you on vitamin C.
- Don't use baking soda when cooking vegetables. (It destroys thiamine and vitamin C.)
- Cook potatoes in their skins.
- Copper pots can destroy vitamin C, folic acid, and vitamin E.

Teenage mothers have greater nutritional needs than women who have already completed their adult growth. Dietary iron is usually low in young women, and the stress of pregnancy can lead to anemia. Also, teenage mothers often have low calcium levels, which if uncorrected can endanger both mother and baby.

TEENAGE MOTHER'S DIET SHOULD INCLUDE AT LEAST SOME:

Liver, meat, egg yolks, asparagus, oatmeal, milk, cheese, green vegetables, dried beans, salmon, sardines.

5. Increased needs during pregnancy

During pregnancy, the body's demand for vitamins increases. For example, no matter how happy a woman is about being pregnant, there is always stress involved. Aside from normal physiological stress, worries about whether the child will be healthy or about having enough money to pay the bills, or any number of similar concerns, can take their toll on mother and fetus.

Stress can cause morning sickness, pregnancy fatigue, headaches, and insomnia.

The body responds to stress by producing more adrenal hormones. These provide the extra energy that's necessary when action is called for. But if there's no physical outlet for the energy, its's redirected to the digestive or nervous system or some other organ system. In many instances, this is what's responsible for pregnancy fatigue, headaches, insomnia, and morning sickness. But what's more important, this sort of adrenal hormone production accelerates the metabolism to such a degree that stores of valuable calcium are depleted, along with protein, phosphorus, and potassium, which are rapidly excreted just when the growing fetus needs them most.

PREGNANT WOMEN NEED A MINIMUM OF:

Daily Requirement

During Pregnancy		*For Nursing Mothers*
74–76 g. protein daily		add 10
1,000 IU	Vitamin A	add 200
400–500 IU	Vitamin D	same
80–100 IU	Vitamin E	add 10
80–100 mg.	Vitamin C	add 20
1.5 mg.	Vitamin B_1	add 0.1 mg.
1.5 mg.	Vitamin B_2	add 0.2 mg.
2.6 mg.	Vitamin B_6	add 0.1 mg.
8–10 mcg.	Vitamin B_{12}	same
800 mcg.	Folic Acid	subtract 300 mcg.
16 mg.	Niacin	add 3 mg.
1,200 mg.	Calcium*	same
1,200 mg.	Phosphorus	same
450 mg.	Magnesium	same
30–60 mg.	Supplemental iron	same
175 mcg.	Iodine	add 25 mcg.
20 mg.	Zinc	add 5 mg.

*Don't use calcium tablets as a replacement for milk unless directed to do so by a doctor.

A good general supplement regimen for prospective, pregnant, and nursing mothers would be:

- High potency multiple vitamin and mineral (be sure that it includes ample amounts of vitamins, A, B_6, C, and folic acid) taken morning and evening with meals.
- Multiple chelated mineral supplement, rich in calcium (two tablets should equal 1,000 mg. calcium and 500 mg. magnesium) taken morning and evening with meals.
- Folic acid, 800 mcg. two times daily.

REMEMBER:

- Many doctors prescribe adequate prenatal multivitamins; check with your physician to avoid doubling up unnecessarily.
- Vitamins are not substitutes for protein or for any other nutrient, or even for one another.
- You can't stop eating and expect vitamins to keep you healthy.

6. What mothers-to-be should know about drugs

The placenta transports nutrients, oxygen, and essential hormones from mother to child, and it passes wastes from baby to mother for elimination. It can also pass drugs taken by the mother to the fetus.

Some drugs, such as insulin, heparin, protamine, and succinylcholine, are molecularly too large to cross the placental membrane. But many others aren't, and some of those can endanger the child. Be sure to check with your doctor on all medications.

DRUGS THAT CAN ENDANGER AN UNBORN CHILD:

Amethopterin	Chloramphenicol
Aminopterin	Chloroquine
Ammonium chloride	Chlorpromazine
Androgens	Chlorpropamide
Barbiturates	Cortisone
Bishydroxycoumarin	Cyclophosphamide
Bromides	Cyclopropane
Busulfan	Estrogens
Chloral hydrate (large doses)	Heroin
Chlorambucil	Iodides

DRUGS THAT CAN ENDANGER AN UNBORN CHILD:

Levorphanol	Quinine
Lithium carbonate	Reserpine
Lysergic acid diethylamide (LSD)	Salicylates
	Smallpox vaccine
Mepivicaine	Sodium warfarin
Methadone	Streptomycin
Methimazole	Sulfonamides
Methotrexate	Sulfonylureas
Nicotine (smoking)	Tetracyclines
Nitrofurantoin	Thalidomide
Novobiocin	Thiazides
Oral progestogens	Tolbutamide
Phenmetrazine	Vitamin A
Phenylbutazone	(large doses)
Potassium iodide	Vitamin K analogs
Propylthiouracil	(large doses)

7. Any questions about chapter I?

If a food is said to be rich in nutrients, does that mean it has all the essential vitamins?

No. All vitamins are nutrients—absorbable components of food—but all nutrients aren't vitamins. Vitamins are just *one* of the six classes of nutrients (carbohydrates, proteins, fats, minerals, vitamins, and water) necessary for cell growth, organ function, utilization of food, and energy.

Are some nutrients more important for my child than others?

All nutrients are important for a child's health because they work together. Macronutrients, like carbohydrates, fat, and protein, provide energy—but only when there are sufficient micronutrients, like vitamins and minerals, to release it.

But, yes, nutrients, like pop records, do have a top ten. With the exclusion of water, they are: protein, carbohydrate, fat, vitamin A, vitamin C, thiamine (vitamin B_1), riboflavin (vitamin B_2), niacin, calcium, and iron. As a general rule, if your child is getting ample amounts of these, he's probably getting enough of the others as well.

My 11-year-old daughter is more active than most boys her age, but I see that the vitamin requirements for boys are always higher. Why is this?

There's nothing discriminatory about it. Vitamin requirements aren't based on energy output, capability or intelligence; they're based on size. The fact is that boys between the ages of eleven and eighteen are generally bigger—heavier—than girls of the same age. Weight is the prime determinant for the USRDA's—for protein and calories as well as for vitamins (see sections 54 and 59).

CHAPTER II

The Vitamin Alphabet

8. Let's start with vitamin A

GETTING TO KNOW IT

- Vitamin A is fat soluble, which means that in order for proper absorption to take place in the digestive tract, a child must have sufficient fats and minerals.
- On commercial food labels it might be listed as the additive *beta carotene*.
- There are two forms of vitamin A:
  1) Preformed Vitamin A—called retinol—which is found only in foods of animal origin.
  2) Provitamin A—called carotene—which is found in food of both plant and animal origin.
- Because vitamin A is fat soluble, it can be stored in the child's body and doesn't have to be replenished every day; for the same reason, an oversupply can lead to an unhealthy buildup and hypervitaminosis (see section 66).
- It can be destroyed by certain medicines (see section 169 for medicines that deplete vitamins) and polyunsaturated fatty acids with carotene.

WHAT IT CAN DO FOR YOUR CHILD

- Combat night blindness.
- Aid in the treatment of many children's eye disorders and help improve weak eyesight. (Forms visual purple in the eye.)
- Build resistance to respiratory infections.
- Promote growth, strong bones, healthy hair, skin, teeth, and gums.

- Help cure acne, impetigo, boils, and open ulcers when applied externally.
- Aid in the treatment of hyperthyroidism.

WHAT TO PICK FROM NATURE'S VITAMIN A PANTRY

Retinol—butter, liver, whole milk, cheese, egg yolk
Provitamin A—leafy green vegetables, carrots, sweet potatoes, winter squash, cantaloupe, fortified margarine

HOW MUCH IS ENOUGH?

Age Group	Daily Minimum to Prevent Deficiency	Daily Minimum for Optimum Health
Newborn to 6 mos.	1,400–1,500 IU	same
6 mos. to 1 yr.	2,000 IU	same
1 yr. to 3 yrs.	2,000–2,500 IU	same
4 yrs. to 6 yrs.	2,500–3,300 IU	same
7 yrs. to 10 yrs.	3,300–5,000 IU	same
Boys 11 to 18 yrs.	5,000 IU	same
Girls 11 to 18 yrs.	4,000–5,000 IU	same

HOW MUCH IS TOO MUCH?

More than 18,500 IU daily can produce toxic effects in infants. (See section 66, Hypervitaminosis.)

WHAT PARENTS SHOULD KNOW ABOUT VITAMIN A SUPPLEMENTS

Vitamin A is usually measured in IU (International Units), but it is also found in USP units (United States Pharmacopeia) and RE (Retinol Equivalents).

This supplement is usually available in two forms, one derived from natural fish oil and the other water dispersible. Water-dispersible supplements are generally recommended for anyone intolerant of oil, particularly teenage acne sufferers.

Vitamin A should *not* be taken with mineral oil.

Vitamin A works best with B complex, vitamin D, vitamin E, calcium, phosphorus, and zinc.

Vitamin A helps prevent vitamin C from oxidizing. (*For deficiency diseases, symptoms, and warning signals, see section* 64.)

9. Vitamin B₁ (Thiamine)

GETTING TO KNOW IT

- Like all the B-complex vitamins, thiamine is water soluble, which means that any excess is excreted and not stored in the child's body. This also means it must be replaced daily.
- On commercial food labels, vitamin B₁ might be listed as the additive *thiamine hydrochloride* or *thiamine mononitrate*.
- Need for this vitamin increases during periods of stress, including those caused by illness and surgery.
- B vitamins are more potent when taken together than when used separately. Because they are synergistic, B₁, B₂, and B₆ should be equally balanced.
- An oversupply of any one B vitamin can increase a child's need for the others.
- Thiamine is easily destroyed by cooking heat, food-processing methods, certain medicines (see section 169 for medicines that deplete vitamins), as well as caffeine, alcohol, and water.

WHAT IT CAN DO FOR YOUR CHILD

- Promote normal appetite.
- Aid in digestion, especially of carbohydrates.
- Help fight car, air, or seasickness.
- Keep nervous system, muscles, and heart functioning normally.
- Improve mental attitude.

WHAT TO PICK FROM NATURE'S VITAMIN B₁ PANTRY

Whole grains, oatmeal, pork, liver, legumes, peanuts, bran, dried yeast.

HOW MUCH IS ENOUGH?

Age Group	Daily Minimum to Prevent Deficiency	Daily Minimum for Optimum Health
Newborn to 6 mos.	.3–.5 mg.	same
6 mos. to 1 yr.	.5–.7 mg.	same
1 yr. to 3 yrs.	.7 mg.	same
4 yrs. to 6 yrs.	.9–1.5 mg.	2.0 mg.
7 yrs. to 10 yrs.	1.2–1.5 mg.	3.0
Boys 11 to 18 yrs.	1.4–1.5 mg.	5–10 mg.
Girls 11 to 18 yrs.	1.1–1.5 mg.	5–10 mg.

HOW MUCH IS TOO MUCH?

No toxicity is known for this water-soluble vitamin because any excess is excreted in the urine and not stored in a child's tissues or organs.

Rare excess symptoms include tremors, nervousness, rapid heartbeat, and allergies.

WHAT PARENTS SHOULD KNOW ABOUT VITAMIN B_1 SUPPLEMENTS

Vitamin B_1 is measured in milligrams (mg.).

It is most effective in a B-complex formula, balanced with B_2 and B_6. It is most effective when the formula contains pantothenic acid, folic acid, and B_{12}.

(*For deficiency diseases, symptoms, and warning signals, see section 64.*)

10. Vitamin B_2 (Riboflavin)

GETTING TO KNOW IT

- An easily absorbed water-soluble vitamin.
- Like the other B vitamins, riboflavin is not stored in a child's body and must be replaced regularly through whole foods or supplements.
- The amount excreted depends on bodily needs and may be accompanied by a protein loss.
- It is the vitamin most Americans are deficient in.
- Unlike thiamine, riboflavin is *not* destroyed by heat, oxidation, or acid. But B_2 does dissolve in cooking liq-

- uids, and it is destroyed by light—especially ultra-violet light. (Opaque milk cartons now protect riboflavin, which used to be destroyed in clear-glass milk bottles.)
- A child's need for this vitamin increases in stress situations.

WHAT IT CAN DO FOR YOUR CHILD

- Promote growth, healthy skin, hair, and nails.
- Alleviate eye fatigue.
- Function with other substances to metabolize carbohydrates, fats, and proteins for the release of energy from food.
- Help eliminate sore mouth, lips, and tongue.

WHAT TO PICK FROM NATURE'S VITAMIN B_2 PANTRY

Liver, milk, yogurt, cottage cheese, leafy green vegetables, fish, kidney.

HOW MUCH IS ENOUGH?

Age Group	Daily Minimum to Prevent Deficiency	Daily Minimum for Optimum Health
Newborn to 6 mos.	.4–.6 mg.	same
6 mos. to 1 yr.	.6–.8 mg.	same
1 yr. to 3 yrs.	.8 mg.	same
4 yrs. to 6 yrs.	1.0–1.7 mg.	3.0 mg.
7 yrs. to 10 yrs.	1.4–1.7 mg.	5.0 mg.
Boys 11 to 14 yrs.	1.6–1.7 mg.	5.0 mg.
Boys 15 to 18 yrs.	1.7 mg.	5.0 mg.
Girls 11 to 14 yrs.	1.3–1.7 mg.	5.0 mg.
Girls 15 to 18 yrs.	1.3–1.7 mg.	5.0 mg.

HOW MUCH IS TOO MUCH?

There are no known toxic effects from this vitamin.

Possible symptoms of minor excess include itching, numbness, and prickling sensations.

WHAT PARENTS SHOULD KNOW ABOUT
VITAMIN B₂ SUPPLEMENTS

Vitamin B_2 is measured in milligrams (mg.).

It is most effective when in a balanced complex with the other B vitamins.

(*For deficiency diseases, symptoms, and warning signals, see section* 64.)

11. Vitamin B₆ (Pyridoxine)

GETTING TO KNOW IT

- A water-soluble vitamin, which is excreted by a child within eight hours after ingestion and, like the other B vitamins, needs to be replaced by whole foods or supplements.
- It must be present for the production of antibodies and red blood cells.
- On commercial food labels, B_6 might be listed as the additive *pyridoxine hydrochloride*.
- It is essential for the proper absorption of vitamin B_{12}.
- It is actually a group of substands—pyridoxine, pyridoxinal, and pyridoxamine—that function together and are necessary for the production of hydrochloric acid, magnesium, and protein metabolism.
- It can be destroyed by long storage, canning, roasting or stewing of meat, water, food-processing techniques, alcohol, and certain medicines. (See section 169 for medicines that deplete vitamins.)

WHAT IT CAN DO FOR YOUR CHILD

- Help prevent various nervous and skin disorders.
- Alleviate nausea—car sickness, air sickness, or seasickness.
- Properly assimilate the protein and fat in the child's diet.
- Work as a natural diuretic.
- Reduce leg cramps.

WHAT TO PICK FROM NATURE'S VITAMIN B₆ PANTRY

Meat, poultry, fish, shellfish, wheat bran, wheat germ, liver, kidney, cantaloupe, cabbage, blackstrap molasses, and milk.

HOW MUCH IS ENOUGH?

Age Group	Daily Minimum to Prevent Deficiency	Daily Minimum for Optimum Health
Newborn to 6 mos.	.3–.4 mg.	same
6 mos. to 1 yr.	.6 mg.	same
1 yr. to 3 yrs.	.7–.9 mg.	same
4 yrs. to 6 yrs.	1.3–2 mg.	same
7 yrs. to 10 yrs.	1.6–2 mg.	3.0 mg.
Boys 11 yrs. to 14 yrs.	1.8–2 mg.	5–10 mg.
Boys 15 yrs. to 18 yrs.	2 mg.	5–10 mg.
Girls 11 yrs to 14 yrs.	1.8–2 mg.	5–10 mg.
Girls 15 yrs. to 18 yrs.	2 mg.	5–10 mg.

Ironically, the requirement for vitamin B_6 is increased if your child is on a high-protein diet.

HOW MUCH IS TOO MUCH?

There are no known toxic effects from B_6.

Possible symptoms of an oversupply are too vivid dream recall and night restlessness.

WHAT PARENTS SHOULD KNOW ABOUT VITAMIN B_6 SUPPLEMENTS

Vitamin B_6 is measured in milligrams (mg.).

To prevent deficiencies in the other B vitamins, B_6 should be taken in equal amounts with B_1 and B_2.

The B vitamins can be purchased in time-disintegrating formulas that provide for gradual release up to ten hours.

Vitamin B_6 might decrease a diabetic's requirement for insulin, and if the dosage is not adjusted, a low-blood-sugar reaction may result.

(*For deficiency diseases, symptoms, and warning signals, see section 64.*)

12. Vitmain B_{12} (Cobalamin)

GETTING TO KNOW IT

- Another water-soluble member of the B family and effective in very small doses.

- It is commonly known as the "red vitamin."
- On commercial food labels, B_{12} might be listed as the additive *cobalamin concentrate* or *cyanocobalamin*.
- To properly benefit a child, this vitamin needs to be combined with calcium during absorption. It is *not* well assimilated through the stomach.
- A poorly functioning thyroid gland impairs B_{12} absorption.
- It can be destroyed by acids and alkalies, water, sunlight, alcohol, and certain medicines. (See section 169 for medicines that deplete vitamins.)

WHAT IT CAN DO FOR YOUR CHILD

- Promote growth and increase appetite.
- Improve concentration, memory, and balance.
- Prevent anemia by forming and regenerating red blood cells.
- Properly utilize fats, carbohydrates, and protein, and thereby provide more energy.
- Decrease irritability by maintaining a healthy nervous system.

WHAT TO PICK FROM NATURE'S VITAMIN B_{12} PANTRY

Liver, beef, pork, fish, shellfish, milk, eggs, cheese, kidney.

HOW MUCH IS ENOUGH?

Age Group	Daily Minimum to Prevent Deficiency	Daily Minimum for Optimum Health
Newborn to 6 mos.	.5–2 mcg.	same
6 mos. to 1 yr. ·	1.5–2 mcg.	same
1 yr. to 3 yrs.	2–3 mcg.	same
4 yrs. to 6 yrs.	2.5–6 mcg.	10 mcg.
7 yrs. to 10 yrs.	3–6 mcg.	10 mcg.
Boys 11 yrs. to 18 yrs.	3–6 mcg.	10 mcg.
Girls 11 yrs. to 18 yrs.	3–6 mcg.	10 mcg.

Keep in mind that a diet low in B_1 and high in folic acid (such as a vegetarian diet) often hides a B_{12} deficiency.

Symptoms of B_{12} deficiency may take more than five years to appear after the child's body supply has been depleted.

Kids on high-protein diets may need extra amounts of B_{12}.

HOW MUCH IS TOO MUCH?

There have been no cases reported of vitamin B_{12} toxicity, even on megadose regimens.

WHAT PARENTS SHOULD KNOW ABOUT
VITAMIN B_{12} SUPPLEMENTS

Vitamin B_{12} works in small doses and is measured in micrograms (mcg.).

Vitamin B_{12} works best with all other B vitamins, as well as vitamins A, E, and C.

(For deficiency diseases, symptoms, and warning signals, see section 64.)

13. Vitamin B_{13} (Orotic Acid)

GETTING TO KNOW IT

- It is a water-soluble B vitamin that metabolizes folic acid and vitamin B_{12}.
- It can be destroyed by water and sunlight.

WHAT IT CAN DO FOR YOUR CHILD

- Aid in the treatment of multiple sclerosis.

WHAT TO PICK FROM NATURE'S VITAMIN B_{13} PANTRY

Root vegetables, whey, the liquid portion of soured or curdled milk.

HOW MUCH IS ENOUGH?

No RDA or USRDA has been established.

HOW MUCH IS TOO MUCH?

Too little is known about the vitamin at present to establish guidelines, but it is not generally recommended for children.

WHAT PARENTS SHOULD KNOW ABOUT
VITAMIN B_{13} SUPPLEMENTS

Vitamin B_{13} is not readily available in the United States, but can be obtained in Europe. It is dispensed as calcium orotate, and should be given to children only under the direction of a physician.

(Deficiency diseases, symptoms and warning signals related to this vitamin are still uncertain.)

14. B_{15} (Pangamic Acid)

GETTING TO KNOW IT

- Water soluble, but because its essential requirement for diet has not been proved, it is not a vitamin in the strict sense.
- Works much like vitamin E in that it is an antioxidant (prevents another substance from oxidation).
- It can be destroyed by water and sunlight.

WHAT IT CAN DO FOR YOUR CHILD

(U.S. research in the case of B_{15} has been limited. The list of benefits given here is based on my study of Soviet tests.)
- Protect against pollutants in urban areas.
- Stimulate immunity responses.
- Relieve some symptoms of asthma.
- Lower blood cholesterol levels.

WHAT TO PICK FROM NATURE'S VITAMIN B_{15} PANTRY

Whole grains, brewer's yeast, pumpkin seeds, whole brown rice, sesame seeds.

HOW MUCH IS ENOUGH?

No RDA or USRDA has been established yet, so check with physician before giving any vitamin B_{15} to a child.

HOW MUCH IS TOO MUCH?

There have been no reported cases of toxicity, but some young athletes have experienced nausea on beginning a B_{15} regimen.

WHAT PARENTS SHOULD KNOW ABOUT
VITAMIN B$_{15}$ SUPPLEMENTS

B$_{15}$ is measured in milligrams (mg.) and works best when taken after the day's largest meal. Consult a nutritionally oriented pediatrician (see section 171) regarding proper dosage for your child.

(*Deficiency diseases, symptoms, and warning signals related to this vitamin are still uncertain.*)

15. Vitamin B$_{17}$ (Laetrile)

GETTING TO KNOW IT

- One of the most controversial "vitamins" of the century.
- A B vitamin made from apricot pits.
- Basically an amygdalin, a chemical compound of two sugar molecules (benzaldehyde and cyanide).
- The one B vitamin that is not present in brewer's yeast.

WHAT IT CAN DO FOR YOUR CHILD

It is purported to have specific cancer-controlling and preventive properties, but it has been rejected by the Food and Drug Administration because latest tests have found it to be ineffective.

(It is *legal* in only twenty-five states in the United States.)

WHAT TO PICK FROM NATURE'S VITAMIN B$_{17}$ PANTRY

A small amount of laetrile is found in the whole kernels of apricots, apples, cherries, peaches, plums, and nectarines. (But, according to *Nutrition Almanac,* no more than thirty of these should be eaten throughout the day—and *never* all at the same time.)

HOW MUCH IS ENOUGH?

No RDA or USRDA has been established owing to its potentially dangerous cyanide content.

HOW MUCH IS TOO MUCH?

No toxicity levels have been established, but ingestion of more than 1.0 g. at any one time is considered dangerous.

WHAT PARENTS SHOULD KNOW ABOUT
VITAMIN B₁₇ SUPPLEMENTS

In light of the recent FDA studies showing its ineffectiveness in treating cancer, I strongly advise personal research and a consultation with a physician before putting a child on any regimen involving B_{17} for *any* reason. If you want a nutrition-oriented physician and know of none in your area, you might write the International College of Applied Nutrition (Box 386, La Habra, California 90631) for a referral. (See section 171 for other referral agencies.)

(Deficiency diseases, symptoms, and warning signals related to this vitamin are still uncertain.)

16. Biotin (Coenzyme R or Vitamin H)

GETTING TO KNOW IT

- Another water-soluble member of the B-complex family.
- Essential for a child's normal metabolism of fat and protein.
- One of the few vitamins that *can* be synthesized by intestinal bacteria, so a child is not dependent on foods for an adequate supply.
- A vitamin that can be destroyed by raw eggs (raw egg white contains avidin, a protein that prevents biotin absorption), along with food-processing techniques, alcohol, water, and certain medicines. (See section 169 for medicines that deplete vitamins.)

WHAT IT CAN DO FOR YOUR CHILD

- Reduce muscle cramps, often called "growing pains."
- Maintain healthy skin.
- Alleviate eczema and infant dermatitis.
- Promote a healthier scalp and hair.

WHAT TO PICK FROM NATURE'S BIOTIN PANTRY

Beef, liver, egg yolk, milk, kidney, unpolished rice, nuts, fruits, brewer's yeast.

HOW MUCH IS ENOUGH?

Age Group	Daily Minimum to Prevent Deficiency	Daily Minimum for Optimum Health
Newborn to 4 yrs.	150 mcg.	same
4 yrs. to 18 yrs.	300 mcg.	same

HOW MUCH IS TOO MUCH?

There is no known toxicity from biotin.

WHAT PARENTS SHOULD KNOW ABOUT BIOTIN SUPPLEMENTS

Biotin is usually measured in micrograms (mcg.).

A child should get at least 25 mcg. daily if he's on anti-biotics or sulfa drugs.

Biotin works synergistically—and more effectively—with B_2, B_6, niacin, and A.

(*For deficiency diseases, symptoms, and warning signals, see section* 64.)

17. Vitamin C (Ascorbic Acid, Cevitamic Acid)

GETTING TO KNOW IT

- A water-soluble vitamin that children must get from dietary sources. (Most animals synthesize their own vitamin C, but man, apes, and guinea pigs cannot.)
- On commercial food labels, vitamin C might appear as the additive *ascorbic acid* or *sodium ascorbate*.
- Used up more rapidly under stress conditions—emotional and physical.
- Aspirin can triple its rate of excretion.
- Essential in the formation of collagen, the primary constituent of bone, cartilage, and connective tissue, and important for the growth and repair of a child's tissue cells, gums, blood vessels, bones, and teeth.

- Important for the child's absorption of iron.
- It is destroyed by carbon monoxide (so city-dwellers need more), as well as water, cooking, heat, and light.
- Recommended as a preventive for crib death or sudden infant death syndrome (SIDS).

WHAT IT CAN DO FOR YOUR CHILD

- Aid in preventing many types of viral and bacterial infections.
- Reduce effects of many allergy-producing substances. (When vitamin C level decreases, histamine increases.)
- Alleviate prickly heat.
- Benefit the treatment of mononucleosis, colitis, conjunctivitis, bronchitis, athlete's foot, canker sores, worms, and more.
- Act as a natural laxative.
- Prevent scurvy.
- Speed up healing after surgery.
- Decrease blood cholestrol.
- Aid in the treatment and prevention of the common cold.

WHAT TO PICK FROM NATURE'S VITAMIN C PANTRY

Citrus fruits, strawberries, green and leafy vegetables, cantaloupe, green pepper, cauliflower, potatoes, sweet potatoes.

HOW MUCH IS ENOUGH?

Age Group	Daily Minimum to Prevent Deficiency	Daily Minimum for Optimum Health
Newborn to 1 yr.	35 mg.	same
1 yr. to 3 yrs.	40–45 mg.	50–100 mg.
4 yrs. to 6 yrs.	45–60 mg.	100 mg.
7 yrs. to 10 yrs.	45–60 mg.	100 mg.
Boys 11 yrs. to 14 yrs.	50–60 mg.	100–500 mg.
Boys 15 yrs to 18 yrs.	60 mg.	500–1,000 mg.
Girls 11 yrs to 14 yrs.	50–60 mg.	500–1,000 mg.
Girls 15 yrs. to 18 yrs.	60 mg.	500–1,000 mg.

HOW MUCH IS TOO MUCH?

There are no proven toxic effects for high dosages of vitamin C, since the child's body will excrete what it doesn't use. Occasional diarrhea, excess urination, skin rashes, and kidney stones may develop on megadoses. These usually do not occur at levels under several thousand milligrams a day, but if they do, simply cut back the dosage.

WHAT PARENTS SHOULD KNOW ABOUT
VITAMIN C SUPPLEMENTS

Vitamin C is measured in milligrams (mg.).

Because this vitamin is excreted in two to three hours, depending on the quantity of food in the child's stomach, it is better for a child to take five 100 mg. chewable tablets than one 500 mg. tablet. For older children I recommend a time-release table for optimal effectiveness.

Large doses of vitamin C can alter the results of laboratory tests. If your child is to have lab work done and is taking vitamin C, inform the doctor so that no errors will be made in diagnosis. (Vitamin C can mask the presence of blood in stool.)

Testing the urine of a diabetic child for sugar might be inaccurate if the child is taking a lot of vitamin C. (But there are testing kits available that are not affected by vitamin C. Ask your pharmacist or physician.)

As a supplement, vitamin C is available in tablets, capsules, syrups, powders, chewable wafers—in just about every form a vitamin can take.

The best vitamin C supplement is one that contains the complete C complex of bioflavonoids, hesperidin, and rutin. (These are sometimes labeled citrus salts.)

Natural or organic vitamin C, though chemically the same as ascorbic acid, is usually easier for children to digest.

(*For deficiency diseases, symptoms, and warning signals, see section* 64.)

18. Calcium Pantothenate (Pantothenic Acid, Panthenol, Vitamin B₅)

GETTING TO KNOW IT

- Another water-soluble member of the B-complex family.
- Like biotin, pantothenic acid (as it is most commonly called) can be synthesized in the child's body by intestinal bacteria.
- Essential for the proper functioning of the adrenal glands.
- Required for the conversion of fat and sugar to energy.
- Necessary for the manufacturing of antibodies that fight infection.
- It is destroyed by food-processing techniques, heat, canning, caffeine, and sulfa drugs. (See section 169 for medicines that deplete vitamins.)

WHAT IT CAN DO FOR YOUR CHILD

- Reduce adverse and toxic effects of many antibiotics.
- Promote wound healing.
- Prevent fatigue.
- Fight infections by building antibodies.

WHAT TO PICK FROM NATURE'S VITAMIN B₅ PANTRY

Liver, kidney, meats, whole grains, egg yolk, bran, wheat germ, crude molasses, nuts, chicken, green vegetables.

HOW MUCH IS ENOUGH?

Age Group	Daily Minimum to Prevent Deficiency	Daily Minimum for Optimum Health
Newborn to 1 yr.	3 mg.	3 mg.
1 yr. to 3 yrs.	5 mg.	5 mg.
4 yrs. to 10 yrs.	10 mg.	15 mg.
Boys and girls 11 yrs. to 18 yrs.	10 mg.	25 mg.

HOW MUCH IS TOO MUCH?

There are no known toxic effects.

WHAT PARENTS SHOULD KNOW ABOUT
VITAMIN B₅ SUPPLEMENTS

Pantothenic acid is measured in milligrams (mg.).

It comes in most B-complex formulas in a variety of strengths from 10 to 100 mg.

Pantothenic acid can help provide a defense against a foreseeable stress situation—or one that the child is presently involved in.

(*For deficiency diseases, symptoms, and warning signals, see section 64.*)

19. Choline

GETTING TO KNOW IT

- A lipotropic (fat emulsifier) that works with inositol (another B-complex member) to utilize fats and cholesterol.
- One of the few substances that can go directly into the brain cells, choline produces a chemical that aids memory. (A so-called blood-brain barrier ordinarily protects the brain against variations in the daily diet.)
- It can be destroyed by water, food processing, alcohol, and sulfa drugs. (See section 169 for medicines that deplete vitamins.)

WHAT IT CAN DO FOR YOUR CHILD

- Produce a soothing effect and alleviate "twitchiness."
- Help a poor memory and improve learning abilities.
- Control a cholesterol buildup.
- Assist in eliminating poisons and drugs from a child's system by aiding the liver.

WHAT TO PICK FROM NATURE'S CHOLINE PANTRY

Egg yolks, liver, brains, wheat germ, green leafy vegetables.

HOW MUCH IS ENOUGH?

No RDA has yet been established for choline, but it has been estimated that the average diet of adults and children over four years of age contains between 500 and 900 mg. per day.

HOW MUCH IS TOO MUCH?

Although there is no known toxicity for choline, taking massive doses over a long period of time can cause a deficiency of vitamin B_6. (It is always advisable to take B-complex vitamins together.)

WHAT PARENTS SHOULD KNOW ABOUT CHOLINE SUPPLEMENTS

Choline is measured in milligrams (mg.).

An average B-complex supplement contains approximately 50 mg. of choline and inositol.

Six lecithin capsules, which are made from soybeans, contain 244 mg. each of inositol and choline.

Choline seems to increase the body's phosphorus, and since phosphorus and calcium should be kept in balance, a child taking large amounts of lecithin (whose active ingredient is phosphatayl choline) might have increased calcium needs.

(*For deficiency diseases, symptoms, and warning signals, see section 64.*)

20. Vitamin D (Calciferol, Viosterol, Erogesterol, "Sunshine Vitamin")

GETTING TO KNOW IT

- A fat-soluble vitamin, which means it can be stored in a child's body and does not necessarily need daily replenishment.
- Acquired through sunlight or diet. (Ultraviolet sunrays act on the oils of a child's skin to produce the vitamin, which is then absorbed into the body.)
- On commercial baby food labels, Vitamin D often appears as the additive *calciferol, ergocalciferol,* or *cholecalciferol.*
- Smog reduces the effectiveness of vitamin D sunshine rays.
- Once a child's suntan is established, vitamin D production through the skin no longer occurs.
- Mineral oil destroys vitamin D.

WHAT IT CAN DO FOR YOUR CHILD

- Promote strong bones and teeth by properly utilizing calcium and phosphorus.
- Help in the treatment of conjunctivitis.
- Aid in preventing colds when taken with vitamins A and C.

WHAT TO PICK FROM NATURE'S VITAMIN D PANTRY

Sardines, herring, salmon, tuna, milk, dairy products, egg yolk, fish oils, fortified margarine.

HOW MUCH IS ENOUGH?

The RDA for vitamin D has been set at 400 IU for all healthy individuals, including infants, provided their consumption of calcium is adequate. Except for therapeutic reasons, 400 IU daily meets the minimum standards for optimum health in children.

HOW MUCH IS TOO MUCH?

I do not advise giving a child more than 1,000 units a day for an extended period, without seeking medical consultation.

Giving 30,000 IU of vitamin D daily to babies over an extended period can easily produce symptoms of toxicity.

More than 45,000 IU of vitamin D, given daily to children, can be dangerous.

Some signs of toxicity are unusual thirst, sore eyes, itching skin, and urinary urgency. (See section 66, Hypervitaminosis.)

WHAT PARENTS SHOULD KNOW ABOUT VITAMIN D SUPPLEMENTS

Supplements are usually supplied in 400 IU capsules or drops.

Vitamin D works best in a child supplied with ample vitamin A, vitamin C, choline, calcium and phosphorus.

(*For deficiency diseases, symptoms, and warning signals, see section 64.*)

21. Vitamin E (Tocopherol)

GETTING TO KNOW IT

- This is a fat-soluble vitamin composed of compounds called tocopherols—alpha, beta, gamma, delta, epsilon, zeta, eta, and theta—alpha-tocopherol being the most effective.
- Unlike other fat-soluble vitamins, E is stored in the body for a relatively short time, much like B and C.
- Sixty to seventy percent of a child's daily doses are excreted in feces.
- It is an active antioxidant, preventing oxidation of fat compounds as well as that of vitamin A, selenium, two amino acids, and some vitamin C.
- It is destroyed by heat, freezing temperatures, oxygen, food processing, iron, chlorine, and mineral oil. (See section 169 for medicines that deplete vitamins.)
- On commercial food labels, vitamin E might appear as the additive *alpha tocopheryl acetate, alpha tocopheryl acetate concentrate,* or *alpha tocopheryl acid succinate.*

WHAT IT CAN DO FOR YOUR CHILD

- Provide more energy by alleviating fatigue.
- Prevent thick scar formation externally (when applied topically, it is absorbed through the skin) and internally.
- Prevent cell membrane damage.
- Speed up the healing of burns.
- Work as a diuretic and an anticoagulant when necessary.

WHAT TO PICK FROM NATURE'S VITAMIN E PANTRY

Wheat germ, vegetable oils, broccoli, Brussels sprouts, whole-grain cereals, eggs, spinach, soybeans, enriched flour.

HOW MUCH IS ENOUGH?

Age Group	Daily Minimum to Prevent Deficiency	Daily Minimum for Optimum Health
Newborn to 6 mos.	3 IU	same
6 mos. to 1 yr.	4 IU	same
1 yr. to 3 yrs.	5–10 IU	same
4 yrs. to 6 yrs.	6–10 IU	10–15 IU
7 yrs. to 10 yrs.	7–10 IU	10–15 IU
Boys 11 to 18 yrs.	10–30 IU	50–100 IU
Girls 11 to 18 yrs.	8–30	50–100 IU

A child on a diet high in polyunsaturated oils might need additional E.

A child who drinks chlorinated water needs extra E.

HOW MUCH IS TOO MUCH?

Vitamin E is essentially nontoxic, but if a child has a vitamin K deficiency, large doses of vitamin E could make that condition worse by impairing normal blood clotting.

It a child has rheumatic heart disease, any vitamin E supplementation should begin with a low dosage and increase gradually.

WHAT PARENTS SHOULD KNOW ABOUT
VITAMIN E SUPPLEMENTS

Formerly measured by weight, vitamin E is now generally designated according to its biological activity in International Units (IU). With this vitamin 1 IU is the same as 1 mg.

It is available in oil-base or water-soluble form. Children who cannot tolerate oil, or whose skin condition is aggravated by oil, would do better with the water-soluble form.

Vitamin E works best with B complex, inositol, and vitamin C.

Since inorganic iron (ferrous sulfate) destroys vitamin E, the two should not be given together. If a child is taking a supplement containing any ferrous sulfate, the E should be taken at least eight hours before or after.

Ferrous gluconate, peptonate, citrate, or fumerate (organic iron complexes) do *not* destroy E.

(For deficiency diseases, symptoms, and warning signals, see section 64.)

22. Vitamin F (Unsaturated Fatty Acids—Linoleic, Linolenic, and Arachidonic)

GETTING TO KNOW IT

- Fat-soluble and composed of unsaturated fatty acids obtained from foods.
- Helps burn saturated fat when intake is balanced two to one (two unsaturated to one saturated).
- If a child has sufficient linoleic acid, the other two fatty acids can be synthesized.
- Twelve teaspoons of sunflower seeds or eighteen pecan halves can furnish a day's complete supply.
- It can be destroyed by an oversupply of saturated fats, heat, and oxygen.

WHAT IT CAN DO FOR YOUR CHILD

- Promote healthy skin and hair.
- Aid in growth by making calcium available to cells.
- Offer some protection against the harmful effects of X rays.
- Aid in weight reduction by burning saturated fats.

WHAT TO PICK FROM NATURE'S VITAMIN F PANTRY

Vegetable oils (such as linseed, sunflower, safflower, soybean, peanut, and wheat germ), peanuts, sunflower seeds, walnuts, pecans, avocados, almonds.

Although most nuts are fine sources of unsaturated fatty acids, Brazil nuts and cashews are *not*.

HOW MUCH IS ENOUGH?

There are no known toxic effects, but an excess can put unwanted pounds on a child.

WHAT PARENTS SHOULD KNOW ABOUT VITAMIN F SUPPLEMENTS

Vitamin F is measured in milligrams (mg.) and is available in capsules of 100 to 150 mg. strengths.

They are rarely necessary for children, who seem to take to the natural sources readily.

(For deficiency diseases, symptoms, and warning signals, see section 64.)

23. Folic Acid (Folacin)

GETTING TO KNOW IT

- Another water-soluble member of the B complex.
- Vital to the formation of red blood cells.
- High vitamin C intakes increase excretion of folic acid.
- Necessary for utilizing sugar and amino acids.
- Aids in the metabolism of protein and is essential for the division of body cells.
- Folic acid can be destroyed by being stored, unprotected, at room temperature for extended periods.
- When folic acid is deficient, antibodies are also deficient.

WHAT IT CAN DO FOR YOUR CHILD

- Promote better color and healthier-looking skin.
- Help ward off anemia.
- Increase appetite after a debilitating illness.
- Act as a natural analgesic for pain.
- Protect against food poisoning and various intestinal parasites.

WHAT TO PICK FROM NATURE'S FOLIC ACID PANTRY

Deep-green leafy vegetables, carrots, egg yolk, cantaloupe, apricots, pumpkins, beans, avocados, whole wheat and dark rye flour, tortula yeast.

HOW MUCH IS ENOUGH?

Age Group	Daily Minimum to Prevent Deficiency	Daily Minimum for Optimum Health
Newborn to 6 mos.	30–100 mcg.	same
6 mos. to 1 yr.	50–100 mcg.	same
1 yr. to 3 yrs.	50–200 mcg.	same
Boys and girls 4 yrs. to 18 yrs.	400 mcg.	same

A child taking aspirin or sulfa medications need more folic acid.

HOW MUCH IS TOO MUCH?

There are no known toxic effects, but a few children have experienced allergic skin reactions.

WHAT PARENTS SHOULD KNOW ABOUT
FOLIC ACID SUPPLEMENTS

Folic acid is measured in micrograms (mcg.).

If a child is on antiepilepsy medication, folic acid might interfere with it; check with the physician.

If you're giving your child folic acid by itself or in a B complex, be sure to tell this to the doctor if the child is being tested for anemia. The doctor is usually alerted to a B_{12} deficiency by a low hematocrit (measurement of red blood cells), but with a folacin supplement the hematocrit might appear normal.

(*For deficiency diseases, symptoms, and warning signals, see section* 64.)

24. Inositol

GETTING TO KNOW IT

- This water-soluble member of the B-complex family is a lipotropic.
- A child's body contains more inositol than any other vitamin except niacin.
- Combined with choline, it forms lecithin.
- Essential for the metabolization of fats and cholesterol.
- It is an important nutrient for brain cells.
- It is destroyed by water, food processing, alcohol, caffeine, certain medicines. (See section 169 for medicines that deplete vitamins.)

WHAT IT CAN DO FOR YOUR CHILD

- Promote healthy hair.
- Help prevent eczema.
- Aid in the redistribution of body fat.
- Help keep cholesterol levels low.

WHAT TO PICK FROM NATURE'S INOSITOL PANTRY

Liver, dried lima beans, cantaloupe, beef brains, raisins, wheat germ, peanuts, cabbage, brewer's yeast.

HOW MUCH IS ENOUGH?

No RDA or USRDA has yet been established, but it is generally recommended that equal amounts of inositol and choline be consumed. Children on fairly balanced diets consume approximately one-half to one gram of inositol daily. But heavy chocolate eaters and cola drinkers can develop an inositol shortage, since caffeine destroys inositol.

HOW MUCH IS TOO MUCH?

There is no known toxicity for inositol.

WHAT PARENTS SHOULD KNOW ABOUT INOSITOL SUPPLEMENTS

Inositol, like choline, is measured in milligrams (mg.).

Six soybean-based lecithin capsules contain approximately 244 mg. each of inositol and choline.

Supplements are available in powders that mix well with liquids, and most B-complex supplements contain approximately 100 mg. each of inositol and choline.

(*For deficiency diseases, symptoms, and warning signals, see section 64.*)

25. Vitamin K (Menadione)

GETTING TO KNOW IT

- There are three K vitamins. K_1 and K_2 can be formed by natural bacteria in the child's intestines. K_3 is a synthetic. They are all fat-soluble.
- Vitamin K sometimes appears in baby foods and formula as the additive *phytonadione*.
- It is essential in forming the blood-clotting chemical prothrombin.
- It can be destroyed by X rays, air pollution, frozen foods, aspirin, and other medicines. (See section 169 for medicines that deplete vitamins.)

WHAT IT CAN DO FOR YOUR CHILD

- Promote proper blood clotting after cuts, scrapes, or surgery.
- Help in preventing internal bleeding and hemorrhages.

WHAT TO PICK FROM NATURE'S VITAMIN K PANTRY

Yogurt, alfalfa, egg yolk, safflower oil, kelp, fish liver oils, leafy green vegetables, milk.

HOW MUCH IS ENOUGH?

Although there has been no dietary allowance established yet, 300 to 500 mcg. is generally considered an adequate supply. But newborn infants require a larger daily intake to prevent any abnormal bleeding, as in hemorrhagic disease.

If your child has frequent nosebleeds, try increasing K naturally with yogurt.

HOW MUCH IS TOO MUCH?

More than 500 mcg. of synthetic vitamin K is not recommended. (See section 66 for symptoms of hypervitaminosis.)

WHAT PARENTS SHOULD KNOW ABOUT
VITAMIN K SUPPLEMENTS

Vitamn K is measured in micrograms (mcg.).

It is not ordinarily included in multiple-vitamin capsules because the abundance of natural vitamin K makes supplementation unnecessary.

(For deficiency diseases, symptoms, and warning signals, see section 64.)

26. Niacin (Nicotinic Acid, Niacinamide, Nicotinamide)

GETTING TO KNOW IT

- Using the amino acid tryptophan, a child's body can manufacture its own niacin (which is actually a water-soluble B vitamin known as B_3).
- A child who is deficient in B_1, B_2, and B_6 will not be able to produce niacin from tryptophan.

- Essential for the synthesis of sex hormones, cortisone, thryoxin, and insulin.
- Niacin is necessary for a healthy nervous system and brain functions, which can affect a child's behavior and learning abilities.
- It can be destroyed by water, food processing, and certain medicines. (See section 169 for medicines that deplete vitamins.)

WHAT IT CAN DO FOR YOUR CHILD

- Give increased energy through proper utilization of food.
- Alleviate stomachaches by promoting a healthy digestive system.
- Provide healthier-looking skin.
- Reduce symptoms of vertigo in Ménière's syndrome.
- Aid in eliminating bad breath.
- Help heal canker sores.
- Ease some attacks of diarrhea.

WHAT TO PICK FROM NATURE'S NIACIN PANTRY

Liver, lean meat, wheat germ, roasted peanuts, figs and dates, the white meat of poultry, avocados, fish, eggs, whole-wheat products, brewer's yeast.

HOW MUCH IS ENOUGH?

Age Group	Daily Minimum to Prevent Deficiency	Daily Minimum for Optimum Health
Newborn to 6 mos.	6–8 mg.	same
6 mos. to 1 yr.	8 mg.	same
1 yr. to 3 yrs.	9 mg.	same
4 yrs. to 6 yrs.	11–20 mg.	same
7 yrs. to 10 yrs.	16–20 mg.	same
Boys 11 to 14 yrs.	18–20 mg.	25–50 mg.
Boys 15 to 18 yrs.	18–20 mg.	25–50 mg.
Girls 11 to 14 yrs.	15–20 mg.	25–50 mg.
Girls 15 to 18 yrs.	14–20 mg.	25–50 mg.

HOW MUCH IS TOO MUCH?

Niacin is essentially nontoxic, except for an uncomfortable warmth or flushing that might result from doses above 75 mg. (Niacinamide minimizes the flush). Prolonged megadoses of several grams a day, certainly not recommended for children, could cause elevations of blood sugar and yellow jaundice.

WHAT PARENTS SHOULD KNOW ABOUT NIACIN SUPPLEMENTS

Niacin is measured in milligrams (mg.); it is usually included in the better B-complex formulas and multivitamin preparations.

It is available in pill and powder form as niacin or niacinamide. (The difference is that niacin—nicotinic acid—might cause flushing, whereas niacinamide—nicotinamide—will not. Flushing can usually be avoided, though, if the pill is taken on a full stomach.)

(*For deficiency diseases, symptoms, and warning signals, see section* 64.)

27. Vitamin P (C Complex, Citrus Bioflavonoids, Rutin, Hesperidin)

GETTING TO KNOW IT

- Water-soluble and necessary for the proper functioning and absorption of vitamin C.
- It is composed of citrin, rutin, and hesperidin, as well as flavones and flavonols. (Flavonoids are the substances that provide the yellow and orange color in citrus fruits.)
- The prime function of bioflavonoids is to increase capillary strength and regulate absorption. (The P stands for permeability, since the vitamin is often called the capillary permeability factor.)
- Works with vitamin C to keep connective tissues healthy.

WHAT IT CAN DO FOR YOUR CHILD

- Prevent bruising by strengthening the walls of capillaries.
- Help build resistance to infection.
- Aid in preventing and healing bleeding gums.

- Increase the effectiveness of vitamin C.
- Help in the treatment of dizziness owing to inner ear disease.

WHAT TO PICK FROM NATURE'S VITAMIN P PANTRY

The white skin and segment part of citrus fruit—lemons, oranges, grapefruit; apricots; strawberries, buckwheat; cherries; rose hips.

HOW MUCH IS ENOUGH?

No daily allowance has been established, but most nutritionists agree that for every 500 mg. of vitamin C a child should have at least 100 mg. of bioflavonoids.

HOW MUCH IS TOO MUCH?

There is no known toxicity.

WHAT PARENTS SHOULD KNOW ABOUT VITAMIN P SUPPLEMENTS

Vitamin P, which is measured in milligrams (mg.), is usually available in a C complex. The ratio of rutin to hesperidin should be equal, but if it isn't, there should be twice as much rutin.

(For deficiency diseases, symptoms, and warning signals, see section 64.)

28. PABA (Para-aminobenzoic Acid)

GETTING TO KNOW IT

- Water-soluble, a member of the B-complex family, it *can* be synthesized in the body.
- Important for forming folic acid and helps in properly using protein.
- Increases the effectiveness of pantothenic acid (B_5).
- Has valuable sun-screening properties.
- It can be destroyed by water, food processing, alcohol, and certain medicines. (See section 169 for medicines that deplete vitamins.)

WHAT IT CAN DO FOR YOUR CHILD

- Reduce the pain of burns.
- Keep skin healthy and smooth.
- Used as an ointment, it can protect against dangerous sunburn.

WHAT TO PICK FROM NATURE'S PABA PANTRY

Liver, kidney, whole grains, rice, bran, wheat germ, molasses, brewer's yeast.

HOW MUCH IS ENOUGH?

No RDA or USRDA has yet been established.

HOW MUCH IS TOO MUCH?

There are no known toxic effects, but long-term programs of high supplementation are not recommended for adults, and certainly not for children.

WHAT PARENTS SHOULD KNOW ABOUT
PABA SUPPLEMENTS

Because PABA can be synthesized in a child's body, I rarely recommend special supplements. It is usually included in a good B complex, as well as in high-quality multivitamins.

If a child tends to burn easily, PABA can be applied externally as an effective natural ointment.

(*For deficiency diseases, symptoms, and warning signals, see section 64.*)

29. Vitamin T

Yes, there is one, but very little is known about it except that it seems to ward off certain forms of anemia and hemophilia by helping in blood coagulation and the formation of platelets. It is found in sesame seeds and egg yolks. There is no recommended dietary allowance for it, and there are no supplements. Also, there is no known toxicity.

30. Vitamin U

I include this vitamin just so that your children can stump the teacher with it. There's even less known about vitamin U than about vitamin T. It is *alleged* to play an important role in healing ulcers, but medical opinion varies on this. Its prime food source is raw cabbage; no known toxicity exists.

31. Any questions about chapter II?

Can a child develop toxic symptoms by getting too much of one vitamin from a natural food?

It's highly unlikely, unless the child is eating large quantities of one or two foods *only,* and those foods are very rich in vitamins A or D. (I did speak to a woman who told me that she had fed her daughter nothing but carrots, spinach, and milk for several months because she had heard that they were healthy foods. Her daughter's skin turned orange—a symptom of hypervitaminosis A. When she followed the advice to put her daughter back on a normal, balanced diet, the orange color disappeared.) Not only is variety the spice of life, it's the key to good nutrition. By offering your child one or more servings from the four basic food groups (see section 91), you'll never have to worry about toxicity—and you can feel confident that you haven't excluded any important vitamins or minerals from your child's diet.

I've heard that giving a child vitamin C will increase his need for that vitamin. Is this true?

No. Children need vitamin C because, unlike puppies and kittens and most other animals (except apes and guinea pigs), they cannot synthesize vitamin C internally and must get it from foods or supplements. A great variety of foods contain vitamin C, but it's easily destroyed by cooking, heat, light, and certain medicines. For this reason, and because of the health benefits vitamin C offers, the advantages of a supplement far outweigh the disadvantages. My own two children, ages nine and four, take a sugarless chewable C daily.

However, it is true that children on *megadose* regimens would have an increased need for the vitamin if the regimen were *abruptly terminated*. The body would have to readjust and might evidence some temporary withdrawal symptoms. But, as I said, this would happen only on megadose regimens, which should be undertaken only on the recommendation of a doctor.

I've had a bottle of chewable vitamin C in the closet for more than a year. Are the vitamins still effective? Are they safe? How can I tell?

If the bottle has been opened, one year is the natural shelf life. If it has not been opened, it's usually good for two years from the time of purchase. I recommend reading labels because most vitamins now have expiration dates printed on them. If your vitamins don't have the dates, mark them yourself. Keep the vitamins stored away from heat, light, and moisture. Refrigeration is not advised (unless you live in an extraordinarily warm climate); neither are bathroom cabinets because of the exposure of moisture.

The way to tell if the vitamins are still effective is to inspect the tablets. If they have spots on them or an acetic, vinegary smell, they're probably deteriorating and losing their potency. I don't recommend buying more than a year's supply of vitamins at a time.

Ascorbic acid does break down into several different chemicals, some of which are suspected of causing diabetes and kidney stones. If you want to play it safe—and you want the effectiveness of the vitamin C—stick to the one-year-opened and two-years-closed rule.

My daughter is allergic to eggs. Is she missing some important vitamin? What other foods can supply it?

She's missing out on a lot of important vitamins and minerals (Vitamin A, B_1, B_2; niacin, calcium, phosphorus, and potassium, to name a few), and protein as well. But fortunately nature provides alternatives—a glass of milk, a whole-grain cereal, and an orange would cover the important nutrients bases just as effectively.

When my son has a cold, he doesn't eat any nutritious food. I know this is the time he needs vitamins most, but what can I do?

Vitamin C can help his cold and his appetite; make sure he's drinking C-rich natural fruit juices. Also, you can purchase a liquid multivitamin mineral supplement and dissolve it in the juice or in desserts, such as apple sauce or yogurt.

My thirteen-year-old son gets very upset before school exams and ends up doing poorly even when he knows the subject. Are there any foods he can eat the night before—or any supplements he can take—that might help?

You might be able to alleviate his exam jitters with a substance called tryptophan, found in bananas, milk, and turkey, which can also be purchased as a supplement. It's a natural relaxant and should be taken with juice or water—not protein (such as milk)—to be most effective. A tablet or two at bedtime can help him get a good night's sleep and allow him to wake up refreshed and better able to cope with his exams.

My daughter has been taking 100–200 mg. of chewable vitamin C daily since she was six. I recently saw a chart of Recommended Daily Dietary Allowances and was stunned to see that the official requirement was only 45 mg.! Have I been overdosing her? Or was that figure a misprint?

The answer to both questions is no. The Recommended Dietary Allowances (RDA), established by the Food and Nutrition Board of the National Research Council of the Academy of Sciences, are merely *estimates* of nutritional needs necessary to ensure the satisfactory growth of children. They *do not* take into account the inestimable nutrient losses that occur during processing and preparation of foods. They *are not* meant to be optimal intakes; nor are they meant to be recommendations for an ideal diet. Actually, they're not even *average* requirements because they are recommendations intended to meet the needs of hypothetically *healthy* children. And when you stop to think of the pollutants in the air, the additives in children's foods, the junk foods in their diets, and the stresses in their lives, you realize that the RDA certainly isn't dealing with the *average* child today.

The USRDA (United States Recommended Daily Allowances), which were formulated by the Food and Drug Administration as legal standards for food labeling in regard to nutrient content, are based on the RDA and purportedly higher than the basic needs of healthy children; but, again, very few kids fall into that hypothetical category.

Kids differ by wide margins, and their physical abilities to handle stress and illnesses differ also. Speaking for myself and for many other nutritionists, the RDA and USRDA are dishearteningly inadequate. No, you haven't been overdosing your daughter. (Vitamin C is water-soluble and does not build up in the body). You've simply been giving her nutritional ammunition to fight for optimal health in today's world.

CHAPTER III

The Mineral Alphabet

32. Calcium

GETTING TO KNOW IT

- A child's body must have sufficient vitamin D in order for calcium to be absorbed.
- Often listed on baby food labels as one of the following additives: *calcium carbonate, calcium glycerophosphate, calcium phosphate, calcium pyrophosphate,* and *calcium sulfate.*
- Calcim works with phosphorus to create healthy bones and teeth. (Almost all the body's calcium is found in the bones and teeth.)
- There is more calcium in your child's body than any other mineral.
- Calcium helps the body utilize iron and helps nutrient passage through cell walls.
- A good cardiovascular structure depends on the working together of calcium and magnesium.
- It can be prevented from proper absorption by large quantities of fat, oxalic acid (found in chocolate and rhubarb), and phytic acid (found in grains).

WHAT IT CAN DO FOR YOUR CHILD

- Maintain strong bones and healthy teeth.
- Alleviate growing pains.
- Quicken reflexes by aiding the nervous system in impulse transmission.
- Keep the heart beating regularly.
- Alleviate insomnia.
- Provide strength and energy by metabolizing the body's iron.

WHAT TO PICK FROM NATURE'S CALCIUM PANTRY

Milk (and all milk products), all cheeses, soybeans, sardines, salmon, peanuts, sunflower seeds, dried beans, green vegetables.

HOW MUCH IS ENOUGH?

Age Group	Daily Minimum to Prevent Deficiency	Daily Minimum for Optimum Health
Newborn to 6 mos.	360–600 mg.	same
6 mos. to 1 yr.	540–600 mg.	same
1 yr. to 3 yrs.	800 mg.	same
4 yrs. to 10 yrs.	800–1,000 mg.	same
Boys 11 yrs. to 18 yrs.	1,000–1,200 mg.	same
Girls 11 yrs. to 18 yrs.	1,000–12,00 mg.	same

HOW MUCH IS TOO MUCH?

Excessive daily intake of over 2,000 mg. might lead to hypercalcemia. (See vitamin D, section 66.)

WHAT PARENTS SHOULD KNOW ABOUT CALCIUM SUPPLEMENTS

Calcium is measured in milligrams (mg.). Most supplements are available in 100–500 mg. tablets.

Bonemeal is a good source of the mineral, though some nutritionists have found that calcium lactate (a milk sugar derivative) and calcium gluconate (a vegetarian source and more potent than lactate) are easier to absorb.

Most good multivitamin and mineral preparations include calcium. (When calcium is combined with magnesium, the proportion should be twice as much calcium as magnesium).

Dolomite is a natural form of calcium and magnesium and requires no vitamin D for assimilation. (Five dolomite capsules equal 750 mg. of calcium.)

(For deficiency diseases, symptoms, and warning signals, see section 64.)

33. Chlorine

GETTING TO KNOW IT

- It's not just a chemical put in drinking water and swimming pools.
- Working with sodium and potassium in a compound form, it regulates the child's alkaline-acid blood balance.
- It helps the liver to function and clean the body of waste products.

WHAT IT CAN DO FOR YOUR CHILD

- Aid in digestion.
- Keep muscles limber.

WHAT TO PICK FROM NATURE'S CHLORINE PANTRY

Table salt, kelp, olives.

HOW MUCH IS ENOUGH?

No RDA or USRDA has been established, but if your child has an average daily salt intake, he's getting enough.

HOW MUCH IS TOO MUCH?

A daily intake of more than 14 grams is excessive and can cause unpleasant side effects.

WHAT PARENTS SHOULD KNOW ABOUT CHLORINE SUPPLEMENTS

Most good multimineral preparations include it.
(*For deficiency diseases, symptoms, and warning signals, see section 64.*)

34. Chromium

GETTING TO KNOW IT

- A mineral that works with insulin in the metabolism of sugar.

- Assists in supplying protein to where it's needed by a child's body.

WHAT IT CAN DO FOR YOUR CHILD

- Aid in growth.
- Help regulate blood sugar levels.

WHAT TO PICK FROM NATURE'S CHROMIUM PANTRY

Meat, shellfish, chicken, corn oil, clams, brewer's yeast.

HOW MUCH IS ENOUGH?

No RDA or USRDA has been established, but for children from birth to one year, 10–60 mcg. is adequate. In a child over four years of age, it has been estimated that 80 mcg. is sufficient.

HOW MUCH IS TOO MUCH?

There is no known toxicity.

WHAT PARENTS SHOULD KNOW ABOUT CHROMIUM SUPPLEMENTS

Chromium is measured in micrograms (mcg.). It can be found in most good multimineral preparations.
(*For deficiency diseases, symptoms, and warning signals, see section 64.*)

35. Cobalt

GETTING TO KNOW IT

- This mineral must be obtained from a food source.
- A part of vitamin B_{12} that is essential for building red blood cells.

WHAT IT CAN DO FOR YOUR CHILD

- Help prevent anemia.

WHAT TO PICK FROM NATURE'S COBALT PANTRY

Meat, kidney, liver, milk, oysters, clams.

HOW MUCH IS ENOUGH?

No RDA or USRDA has been established, but only *very small* amounts (less than 8 mcg.) are necessary in the diet.

HOW MUCH IS TOO MUCH?

There is no known toxicity.

WHAT PARENTS SHOULD KNOW ABOUT COBALT SUPPLEMENTS

It is rarely found in supplement form.
(*For deficiency diseases, symptoms, and warning signals, see section 64.*)

36. Copper

GETTING TO KNOW IT

- A necessary mineral for converting the iron in a child's body into hemoglobin.
- It is essential for the utilization of vitamin C, and it can reach the bloodstream fifteen minutes after it is ingested.
- It aids the amino acids tyrosine and allows it to work as a pigmenting factor for the skin and hair.
- It is not easily destroyed.
- It is often listed on baby food labels as the additive *copper gluconate* or *cupric sulfate*.

WHAT IT CAN DO FOR YOUR CHILD

- Improve energy and alertness by aiding effective iron absorption.

WHAT TO PICK FROM NATURE'S COPPER PANTRY

Dried beans, peas, whole wheat, prunes, seafood, beef liver.

HOW MUCH IS ENOUGH?

No RDA or USRDA has been set, but the National Academy of Sciences-National Research Council (NAS-NRC) estimated adequate allowance for children from birth to six months is 0.5–0.7 mg., and from six months to one year 0.7–1.0 mg.

HOW MUCH IS TOO MUCH?

No more than 2 mg. are necessary for children over four years of age. Except in cases of abnormal copper metabolism (such as Wilson's disease), toxicity is rare. Only a small amount of this mineral is absorbed; most is excreted.

An excess often causes insomnia and psychological disturbances.

WHAT PARENTS SHOULD KNOW ABOUT COPPER SUPPLEMENTS

Copper is measured in milligrams (mg.). It is often included in multivitamin and mineral supplements in small dosages.

If your child eats enough whole-grain products and/or leafy green vegetables, you don't have to worry about his copper intake. Supplements are rarely necessary.

(For deficiency diseases, symptoms, and warning signals, see section 64.)

37. Fluorine

GETTING TO KNOW IT

- Essentially fluorine is a mineral that works with calcium to strengthen bones and teeth.
- The fluoride that is added to drinking water is sodium fluoride; this is not the same as calcium fluoride, which is natural.
- It cuts down the acid in the mouth, which is caused by carbohydrates, and helps prevent tooth decay.

WHAT IT CAN DO FOR YOUR CHILD

- Help prevent dental caries.
- Aid in the formation of strong bones.

WHAT TO PICK FROM NATURE'S FLUORINE PANTRY

Seafoods, gelatin, fluoridated drinking water.

HOW MUCH IS ENOUGH?

No RDA or USRDA has been established, but most children get about 1 mg. daily from fluoridated drinking water, which is considered safe and adequate by NAS-NRC standards.

HOW MUCH IS TOO MUCH?

Excessive amounts are definitely dangerous. An intake of 20 mg. or more can be toxic. (Calcium is an antidote for fluoride poisoning.)

WHAT PARENTS SHOULD KNOW ABOUT
FLUORINE SUPPLEMENTS

Do not give your child additional fluoride unless it is prescribed by a physician or a dentist.

(For deficiency diseases, symptoms, and warning signals, see section 64.)

38. Iodine (Iodide)

GETTING TO KNOW IT

- The thyroid gland contains most of the body's iodine.
- It is supplied in many commercially prepared foods as *iodized salt*.
- Because iodine influences the thyroid gland, which controls metabolism, an undersupply can cause a child to have slow mental reaction, marked lack of energy, and unexplainable weight gain.

WHAT IT CAN DO FOR YOUR CHILD

- Promote proper growth.
- Improve learning ability.
- Engender more energy and general get-up-and-go.
- Control weight by burning up excess fat.
- Foster healthy hair, nails, teeth, and skin.

WHAT TO PICK FROM NATURE'S IODINE PANTRY

Kelp, onions, all seafood, vegetables grown in iodine-rich soil.

HOW MUCH IS ENOUGH?

Age Group	Daily Minimum to Prevent Deficiency	Daily Minimum for Optimum Health
Newborn to 6 mos.	40–45 mcg.	same
6 mos. to 1 yr.	50 mcg.	same
1 yr. to 3 yrs.	70 mcg.	same
4 yrs. to 6 yrs.	90–150 mcg.	same
7 yrs. to 10 yrs.	120–150 mcg.	same
Boys and girls 11 yrs. to 18 yrs.	150 mcg.	same

HOW MUCH IS TOO MUCH?

There is no known toxicity from natural iodine, but it is possible for large amounts of kelp to cause an overactivity of the thyroid gland.

As a drug, iodine can be harmful if prescribed or taken incorrectly.

WHAT PARENTS SHOULD KNOW ABOUT IODINE SUPPLEMENTS

Iodine is measured in micrograms (mcg.), and very small amounts are necessary. It's often included in multimineral and high-potency vitamin supplements in doses of 0.15 mcg.

Natural kelp is the best source of supplemental iodine. I don't recommend any additional iodine supplements for children unless a doctor prescribes them.

(*For deficiency diseases, symptoms, and warning signals, see section 64.*)

39. Iron

GETTING TO KNOW IT

- A major mineral, it is essential for life: needed for the production of hemoglobin (red blood corpuscles), myoglobin (red pigment in muscles), and certain enzymes.

- Copper, cobalt, manganese, and vitamin C are necessary for the assimilation of iron.
- Menstruating girls lose almost twice as much iron a month as do boys the same age.
- Hemoglobin, which accounts for most of a child's iron, is recycled and reused as blood cells are replaced approximately every one hundred and twenty days.
- Excess phosphorus, as well as substances called phytates in unleavened whole wheat, reduce the availability of iron to the child.
- It often appears on commercial food labels as one of the following additives: *ferric phosphate, iron phosphate, ferric orthophosphate, sodium ferric pyrophosphate, ferric pyrophosphate, iron pyrophosphate, ferrous fumarate, ferrous gluconate, and electrolytic iron.*
- Iron is important for the proper metabolization of B vitamins.

WHAT IT CAN DO FOR YOUR CHILD

- Cure as well as prevent iron-deficiency anemia.
- Increase energy by preventing fatigue.
- Bring back healthy color to the cheeks.
- Aid in growth.
- Promote resistance to disease.

WHAT TO PICK FROM NATURE'S IRON PANTRY

Liver, farina, raw clams, dried peaches, red meat, egg yolks, nuts, asparagus, oatmeal.

HOW MUCH IS ENOUGH?

Age Group	Daily Minimum to Prevent Deficiency	Daily Minimum for Optimum Health
Newborn to 6 mos.	10–15 mg.	same
6 mos. to 1 yr.	15 mg.	same
1 yr. to 3 yrs.	10–15 mg.	same
4 yrs. to 10 yrs.	10–18 mg.	same
Boys and girls 11 yrs. to 18 yrs.	18 mg.	same

HOW MUCH IS TOO MUCH?

Toxicity is rare, but prolonged unnecessary dosages of iron (iron-fortified vitamins) can be hazardous to children. (Iron poisoning has been found in children whose mothers have taken too many iron pills during pregnancy.) Iron should not be given to any child with sickle-cell anemia, hemochromatosis, or thalassemia.

WHAT PARENTS SHOULD KNOW ABOUT IRON SUPPLEMENTS

Iron is measured in milligrams (mg.). It is included in most multivitamin-mineral supplements. Check the label to make sure that the iron in the supplement is organic—ferrous gluconate, ferrous fumerate, ferrous citrate, or ferrous peptonate—and not ferrous sulfate, which is inorganic and can destroy vitamin E, unles the two are taken eight hours apart.

Keep iron supplements out of the reach of children!

(*For deficiency diseases, symptoms, and warning signals, see section 64.*)

40. Magnesium

GETTING TO KNOW IT

- Known as the antistress mineral, magnesium is necessary for calcium and vitamin C metabolism, as well as that of phosphorus, sodium, and potassium.
- It is essential for proper nerve and muscle functioning.
- It is important for converting blood sugar into energy.
- On commercial food labels, it often appears as the additives *magnesium phosphate* or *magnesium sulfate*.
- It can be destroyed by certain medicines. (See section 169 for medicines that deplete vitamins.)

WHAT IT CAN DO FOR YOUR CHILD

- Help relieve stomachaches caused by indigestion.
- Improve moods by warding off depression.
- Promote healthier teeth.
- Improve the cardiovascular system.

WHAT TO PICK FROM NATURE'S MAGNESIUM PANTRY

Figs, lemons, grapefruit, yellow corn, almonds, apples, nuts, seeds, dark-green vegetables.

HOW MUCH IS ENOUGH?

Age Group	Daily Minimum to Prevent Deficiency	Daily Minimum for Optimum Health
Newborn to 6 mos.	50–70 mg.	same
6 mos. to 1 yr.	70 mg.	same
1 yr. to 3 yrs.	150–200 mg.	same
4 yrs. to 6 yrs.	200 mg.	same
7 yrs. to 10 yrs.	250–400 mg.	same
Boys 11 to 14 yrs.	350–400 mg.	same
Boys 15 to 18 yrs.	400 mg.	same
Girls 11 to 14 yrs.	300–400 mg.	same
Girls 15 to 18 yrs.	300–400 mg.	same

Children on high-protein diets have an increased need for magnesium. Also, if calcium intake is high (as with heavy milk drinkers), more magnesium-rich foods should be included in the diet.

HOW MUCH IS TOO MUCH?

Large amounts, over an extended period of time, can be toxic—especially if a child's calcium intake is low and his phosphorus intake is high. In children with kidney problems, there is a greater danger of toxicity because the rate of excretion will be slower.

WHAT PARENTS SHOULD KNOW ABOUT
MAGNESIUM SUPPLEMENTS

Magnesium is measured in milligrams (mg.). It is usually included in multivitamin and mineral preparations. (It is best if these are chelated.)

Dolomite, which has magnesium and calcium in perfect balance (half as much magnesium as calcium), is a fine supplement, if one is necessary.

If your child eats enough nuts, seeds, or green vegetables—

or if you live in an area with hard water—it is most likely that he or she gets ample amounts of magnesium.

(For deficiency diseases, symptoms, and warning signals, see section 64.)

41. Manganese

GETTING TO KNOW IT

- An important mineral for bone structure, proper digestion, and the utilization of food.
- It helps in the formation of thyroxin, the principal hormone of the thyroid gland.
- It's necessary for the body's proper use of biotin, B_1, and vitamin C.
- Large intakes of calcium and phosphorus will inhibit its absorption.

WHAT IT CAN DO FOR YOUR CHILD

- Provide more energy by eliminating fatigue.
- Allow him or her to do better in school by improving memory.
- Aid in quickening muscle reflexes—help him or her become a better pitcher on the softball team.
- Reduce nervous irritability.

WHAT TO PICK FROM NATURE'S MANGANESE PANTRY

Nuts, leafy green vegetables, peas, beets, egg yolks, whole-grain cereals.

HOW MUCH IS ENOUGH?

No RDA or USRDA has yet been set, but the NAS-NRC estimates for newborn to six months are 0.5–0.7 mg., and, from six months to one year, 0.7–1.0 mg. For children four years of age and older, 2.5 to 7.0 mg. has generally been accepted as the daily minimum.

Children who are heavy meat eaters and milk drinkers might need a bit more.

HOW MUCH IS TOO MUCH?

Toxicity is rare, except from industrial sources.

WHAT PARENTS SHOULD KNOW ABOUT
MANGANESE SUPPLEMENTS

Manganese is measured in milligrams (mg.). Most multivitamin and mineral preparations contain it in dosages of 1 to 9 mg.

(For deficiency diseases, symptoms, and warning signals, see section 64.)

42. Molybdenum

GETTING TO KNOW IT

• This trace mineral aids in carbohydrate and fat metabolism and plays an important part in iron utilization.

WHAT IT CAN DO FOR YOUR CHILD

• Help in preventing anemia.

WHAT TO PICK FROM NATURE'S MOLYBDENUM PANTRY

Leafy dark green vegetables, whole grains, legumes.
(The molybdenum content of these foods is completely dependent on the soil content.)

HOW MUCH IS ENOUGH?

No RDA or USRDA has been set, but the NAS-NRC estimates for newborn to six months are 30–60 mcg., and for children from six months to one year, 40–80 mcg.

HOW MUCH IS TOO MUCH?

Toxicity is rare, but a high intake may result in a copper deficiency.

Supplements are not ordinarily available. There is really no need for molybdenum supplementation, unless all the food your child consumes comes from nutrient-deficient soil.

(*No deficiency diseases are known.*)

43. Phosphorus

GETTING TO KNOW IT

- Phosphorus is present in every cell in your child's body and involved in all physiological chemical reactions.
- It is necessary for normal bone and tooth structure, as well as normal heart and kidney functioning.
- Calcium and vitamin D are essential to proper phosphorus functioning. (Calcium and phosphorus should be balanced two to one, with twice as much calcium as phosphorus.)
- It is needed for the proper transference of nerve impulses and adequate niacin assimilation.
- Too much iron or magnesium can make phosphorus ineffective.
- It is included in many commercially prepared foods and listed as the additive *calcium phosphate, sodium phosphate,* or *sodium pyrophosphate*.

WHAT IT CAN DO FOR YOUR CHILD

- Aid in growth and promote healthy gums and teeth.
- Speed up healing of broken bones or other injuries.
- Increase energy for learning or sports by helping in the metabolization of fats and starches.

WHAT TO PICK FROM NATURE'S PHOSPHORUS PANTRY

Fish, poultry, meat, eggs, whole grains, nuts, seeds.

HOW MUCH IS ENOUGH?

Age Group	Daily Minimum to Prevent Deficiency	Daily Minimum for Optimum Health
Newborn to 6 mos.	240–500 mg.	same
6 mos. to 1 yr.	360–500 mg.	same
1 yr. to 3 yrs.	800 mg.	same
4 yrs. to 10 yrs.	800–1,000 mg.	same
Boys and girls 11 yrs. to 18 yrs.	1,000–1,200 mg.	1,000–1,500 mg.

HOW MUCH IS TOO MUCH?

Toxicity is rare, but be on the lookout for foods preserved with phosphates and consider that as part of your child's daily intake.

WHAT PARENTS SHOULD KNOW ABOUT PHOSPHORUS SUPPLEMENTS

Phosphorus is measured in milligrams (mg.). It can be found in bonemeal—a fine natural supplement. (Make sure vitamin D has been added to help assimilation.)

Since the diets of most children are high in phosphorus, supplementation is usually unnecessary. But be aware that too much phosphorus can decrease a child's calcium.

(*For deficiency diseases, symptoms, and warning signals, see section 64.*)

44. Potassium

GETTING TO KNOW IT

- This mineral works with sodium to regulate a child's heart rhythms and water balance.
- An imbalance between sodium and potassium can impair nerve and muscle function.
- It is included in commercially prepared foods and often listed as one of the following additives: *potassium chloride, potassium glycerophosphate,* and *potassium iodide.*
- Hypoglycemia (low blood sugar) is known to cause potassium loss, as does a long fast and severe diarrhea.
- Sugar and diuretics can destroy potassium.

WHAT IT CAN DO FOR YOUR CHILD

- Improve learning ability by sending more oxygen to the brain.
- Alleviate colic.
- Aid in allergy treatments.
- Help reduce blood pressure and sugar levels in diabetic children.
- Help in the proper elimination of body wastes.
- Aid in the treatment of diarrhea.

WHAT TO PICK FROM NATURE'S POTASSIUM PANTRY

Bananas, potatoes, citrus fruits, watercress, sunflower seeds, all leafy green vegetables.

HOW MUCH IS ENOUGH?

No RDA or USRDA has yet been set, but for children over four years of age an intake of 2,000 mg. is considered healthy. (For newborn to one year, 350–1,275 mg. is adequate.)

Keep in mind that stress causes a loss of potassium, as does a heavy intake of sugary junk food.

HOW MUCH IS TOO MUCH?

There is no known toxicity from potassium, but more than 25 g. of potassium chloride can cause toxicity.

WHAT PARENTS SHOULD KNOW ABOUT POTASSIUM SUPPLEMENTS

Potassium is measured in milligrams (mg.). It is available in most high-potency and multivitamin and mineral preparations. Organic potassium (gluconate, citrate, fumerate) is better for a child than inorganic potassium "salts" (sulfate, chloride, oxide, and carbonate).

(*For deficiency diseases, symptoms, and warning signals, see section 64.*)

45. Selenium

GETTING TO KNOW IT

- An antioxidant that works synergistically with vitamin E (which means the two together are stronger than the sum of the equal parts).
- Boys who have reached puberty have a greater need for selenium than do girls. Half of a male's body supply concentrates in the testicles and seminal ducts and is lost in the semen.
- It is easily destroyed by food processing.

WHAT IT CAN DO FOR YOUR CHILD

- Improve oxygen utilization, helping heart and lungs.
- Help in the treatment and prevention of dandruff.
- Possibly neutralize certain carcinogens that are ingested from foods. (New studies show that it can prevent the spread of some existing tumors.)
- Provide elasticity in tissues and muscles for young athletes.

WHAT TO PICK FROM NATURE'S SELENIUM PANTRY

Wheat germ, bran, tuna fish, onions, tomatoes, broccoli.

HOW MUCH IS ENOUGH?

No RDA or USRDA has yet been established, but for newborn to six months, the adequate intake is 10–40 mcg.; from six months to one year, it's 20–60 mcg. Children over four years of age need 50–100 mcg.

HOW MUCH IS TOO MUCH?

It is not advisable to exceed 200 mcg. daily. Selenium can be toxic in its pure form.

WHAT PARENTS SHOULD KNOW ABOUT SELENIUM SUPPLEMENTS

Selenium is available in small microgram doses, but natural foods supply sufficient amounts when eaten regularly. I would not advise selenium supplements for children under ordinary circumstances.

(*For deficiency diseases, symptoms, and warning signals, see section 64.*)

46. Sodium

GETTING TO KNOW IT

- Sodium aids in keeping calcium and other minerals soluble in the blood.
- With potassium, sodium regulates muscle contraction and nerve stimulation as well as the balance of water in a child's body.
- It is necessary for production of hydrochloric acid in the stomach.
- In commercially prepared foods, sodium is often listed on the label as iodized salt.

WHAT IT CAN DO FOR YOUR CHILD

- Prevent heat prostration or sunstroke after hard play on a hot day.
- Help keep reflexes toned and functioning.

WHAT TO PICK FROM NATURE'S SODIUM PANTRY

Salt, shellfish, beets, grains, bacon, kidney, kelp.

HOW MUCH IS ENOUGH?

No RDA or USRDA has been established, but it is suggested that a single gram of sodium chloride (salt) for each kilogram of water drunk is sufficient.

HOW MUCH IS TOO MUCH?

More than 13 g. of sodium chloride daily can produce toxic effects.

Keep in mind that most fast foods that children eat are heavily oversalted (see section 102), and that excessive salt in food interferes with proper utilization of nourishing protein foods.

WHAT PARENTS SHOULD KNOW ABOUT
SODIUM SUPPLEMENTS

Basically, they're unnecessary for children. (Kelp is about the best natural supplement.)

If your child has been told to cut down on salt because of high blood pressure or for other reasons, be sure to check the labels of the foods you buy. Look for *salt, sodium,* or the chemical symbol *Na;* avoid luncheon meats, frankfurters, salted cured meats, as well as ketchup, chili sauce, soy sauce, and mustard. Also, avoid using baking powder or baking soda in cooking.

(*For deficiency diseases, symptoms, and warning signals, see section 64.*)

47. Sulfur

GETTING TO KNOW IT

- Sulfur works with B-complex vitamins for basic body metabolism, and it is part of the tissue-building amino acids.
- It aids the liver in bile secretion and helps maintain the oxygen balance required for proper brain function.
- It is often called nature's beauty mineral.

WHAT IT CAN DO FOR YOUR CHILD

- Keep skin clear and smooth and make hair more lustrous.
- Help fight bacterial infections.

WHAT TO PICK FROM NATURE'S SULFUR PANTRY

Cabbage, dried beans, fish, lean beef, eggs, nuts.

HOW MUCH IS ENOUGH?

No RDA or USRDA has been set, but any diet with ample protein will be sufficient in sulfur.

HOW MUCH IS TOO MUCH?

There is no known toxicity from organic sulfur, but inorganic sulfur in large amounts can be hazardous to a child's health.

Sulfur is neither readily available nor in any way necessary as a supplement for a child. It can be found, though, as a topical ointment or cream and can be used effectively for skin problems. (*No deficiency disease or symptoms are known.*)

48. Vanadium

All you need to know about vanadium is that it is a trace mineral that essentially inhibits the formation of cholesterol in blood vessels. There are no known deficiencies of it, no supplements for it, but it can be easily toxic if taken in synthetic form. It is found in fish, and a good fish dinner is all a child needs for an adequate supply.

49. Zinc

GETTING TO KNOW IT

- Zinc is what I call a major mineral. It's a traffic police-man in the body, directing and overseeing the efficient maintenance of enzyme systems and cells and the uninhibited flow of body process.
- It helps in the formation of insulin and is essential for protein synthesis.
- It is important for maintaining the child's acid-alkaline balance and governs the contractability of his muscles.
- It is vital in the development of all reproductive organs.
- In commercially prepared foods it is listed as the additive *zinc oxide* or *zinc sulfate*.
- Recent studies have indicated its importance in brain function and the treatment of schizophrenia.
- Food processing destroys zinc, and many foods are low in it because they're grown in nutrient-deficient soil.

WHAT IT CAN DO FOR YOUR CHILD

- Get rid of white spots on the fingernails
- Improve learning aptitude by increasing mental alertness.
- Decrease cholesterol.

- Promote a better appetite by improving ability to taste.
- Accelerate healing time for scrapes, cuts, and internal wounds.
- Promote growth.

WHAT TO PICK FROM NATURE'S ZINC PANTRY

Lamb chops, pork, wheat germ, round steak, pumpkin seeds, sunflower seeds, eggs, ground mustard, brewer's yeast, nonfat dry milk.

HOW MUCH IS ENOUGH?

Age Group	Daily Minimum to Prevent Deficiency	Daily Minimum for Optimum Health
Newborn to 6 mos.	3–5 mg.	same
6 mos. to 1 yr.	5 mg.	same
1 yr. to 3 yrs.	8–10 mg.	same
4 yrs. to 6 yrs.	10–15 mg.	same
7 yrs. to 10 yrs.	10–15 mg.	same
Boys and girls 11 yrs. to 18 yrs.	15 mg.	same

Diabetic children and children taking large amounts of vitamin B_6 need higher intakes of zinc.

HOW MUCH IS TOO MUCH?

Doses over 100 mg. are not recommended. It is virtually nontoxic, except when there is an excessive intake and the food ingested has been stored in galvanized containers.

Large doses taken over an extended period can decrease copper levels, which in turn can lead to anemia and abnormal heart rhythms.

WHAT PARENTS SHOULD KNOW ABOUT ZINC SUPPLEMENTS

Zinc, which is measured in milligrams (mg.), is available in all good multivitamin and multimineral preparations.

It is available as *zinc sulfate* or *zinc gluconate*; both are effective, but the latter has been found to be more easily tolerated.

As a supplement, chelated zinc seems to work better.

(*For deficiency diseases, symptoms, and warning signals, see section 64.*)

50. Any questions about chapter III?

My eleven-year-old daughter is maturing very rapidly, but I've noticed that her hair has lost its luster and her skin has become dry. She takes a vitamin pill every morning (because she eats a lot of junk food), but I think it's minerals that she needs. What would you suggest?

The first thing would be to get her off junk food (see section 103), then make sure that fish, wheat germ, yeast, and liver are included in her diet. Skin cannot repair itself, but a tablespoon of cod liver oil (flavored) can help dry skin. Vitamins A and D are important for a good complexion. Hair, on the other hand, can repair itself, and with the aid of vitamin A and the B-complex vitamins—especially biotin, inositol, pantothenic acid, folic acid, and PABA—even formerly dry hair can become lustrous.

Zinc is an antistress mineral, and combined with vitamin B complex and C, it can help counteract the stress that your child's body is incurring with maturation and has already incurred from excessive consumption of carbohydrates, refined sugars, and caffeine (which is present in colas, other soft drinks, chocolate, and cocoa, as well as in some RX and many over-the-counter drugs). Caffeine may be robbing your child of inositol, which is needed for healthy hair.

For her hair I would suggest a multimineral supplement; but because of her skin problem, there should be no iodine included in the supplement. Iodine has been known to worsen certain skin conditions. For this reason, you might want to cut down on her intake of iodized salt.

My son has a taste for plain salt. (He'll just pour it out of the shaker into his mouth). Does this indicate a deficiency?

Possibly. Your son's diet may be too rich in potassium (tomato juice, bananas, potatoes, citrus fruits, all leafy green vegetables, and sunflower seeds). There is a sodium-potassium balance; too much of one can cause a deficiency of the other.

If he is overconsuming one potassium-rich food, that might account for his salt hunger.

Do white spots on a child's fingernails signify some sort of calcium deficiency?

No, they more likely indicate a zinc deficiency. Make sure you include meats (rare steaks, lamb chops, and pork loin) in your child's diet, along with wheat germ, brewer's yeast, and eggs. Nonfat dry milk, pumpkin seeds, and oysters are also good suppliers of zinc. If you feel you can't organize his diet to include these foods regularly, you might want to try a multiple mineral supplement with at least 15 mg. of zinc.

If your child's nails are also thin or weak, this could indicate a general low-protein intake. Ridges on the nails are often clues to a lack of B_6 and other B-complex vitamins in the diet. Calcium will toughen nails, and choline in 1-g.-per-day doses (for a child over four years of age) can help keep them strong.

CHAPTER IV

A Child's Garden of Nutrition— Water, Protein, Carbohydrates, Fats, and More

51. Water

Everything in a child's garden of nutrition needs water to grow—especially the child. Although it provides no calories or vitamins, water is a nutrient that no child can live without.

Babies, as mothers have always suspected from those mounting piles of diapers, are 60 percent water. This is in constant need of replenishment, since infants lose a great amount of body water, not only through urine but also through stools and perspiration. And because they are more susceptible to vomiting and diarrhea, which incur heavy water losses, they must be supplied ample amounts to avoid dehydration.

> *A child can live weeks without food—but only a few days without water.*

Although the fluid in breast milk and formula can ordinarily satisfy a baby's need, it is wise to offer a few ounces of water (without sugar) between meals—especially in hot weather or when the infant is ill. (It's best to boil the water for the baby's first year. Be sure to *cool it* before giving it to baby.)

Water is the basic solvent for all the products of digestion; it keeps all your child's bodily processes functioning. It is essential for removing wastes and regulating the body's normal temperature.

All drinkable liquids can substitute for your child's daily water requirement. (Six glasses a day for a child over four years of age is the usual recommendation.) If you're traveling and liquids aren't available, most fruits, which have a high water content (and are a lot less messy in a car on a bumpy road), can be substituted.

As safe and wonderful as water is, you should be aware that, as with all things used to excess, too much can be dangerous. One and a half gallons (that's sixteen to twenty-four glasses) in about an hour could be dangerous to an adult—and could kill an infant.

52. Protein—the Superstar Nutrient

Proteins are used by your child's body to build new tissue and repair damaged cells. They're also used to make hormones, enzymes, keep the acid-alkaline blood content balanced, and take out the garbage, among other things.

As protein is digested, it is broken down into smaller compounds called amino acids. When these amino acids reach the cells of your child's body, they're formed into protein again. It's a marvelous cycle.

Though the same twenty amino acids form all proteins (and there are thousands of them), they each perform a different function in a different area of the body.

> *All proteins are nutrients, but—wonderful as they are—they're not all equal.*

Proteins can be divided into two classes—complete and incomplete. Complete protein provides the proper balance of necessary amino acids. Incomplete protein lacks certain essential amino acids and is not used efficiently when eaten alone. However, when small amounts of complete (animal source) protein are combined with incomplete protein, the combination can give your child better nutrition than either one alone.

The following are lists of some complete and incomplete protein foods. Mix and match them in breakfasts, lunches, and dinners, and you can be sure your child will be getting the best in protein nourishment.

COMPLETE PROTEIN

Type of Food	Serving Size	Protein Content
Cheese		
American	1 slice (1 oz.)	6.6 g.
cheddar	1 slice (Longhorn style)	6.0 g.
cottage	½ cup (large curd)	15.3 g.
	½ cup (small curd)	14.3 g.
Swiss	1 slice (1 oz.)	7.8 g.
Eggs		
extra large	1	7.4 g.
large	1	6.5 g.
medium	1	5.7 g.
Fish		
cod	1 (5-in.) fillet	18.5 g.
flounder	1 (6-in.) fillet	17.1 g.
salmon (broiled)	1 oz.	7.7 g.
tuna	1 can (3½ oz.) solid	27.7 g.
	1 can (3½ oz.) chunk	25.8 g.
Meat		
frankfurter	1	7.1 g.
ham	1 (3 oz.) slice	19.6 g.
hamburger	1 (4 oz.) patty (cooked)	23.4 g.
lamb chop	1 (3.4 oz.) chop	20.9 g.
liver (beef)	1 (3 oz.) slice	119.8 g.
liver (chicken)	1 liver	6.6 g.
pork chop	1 (3 oz.) chop	20.8 g.
roast beef	3 oz. (rump roast)	20.1 g.
Milk		
whole	1 cup	8.5 g.
skim	1 cup	8.8 g.
powdered	1 cup	33.8 g.
yogurt	1 cup (made from whole milk)	7.4 g.
	(made from skim milk)	8.3 g.
Poultry		
chicken (cooked-fried)	1 wing	8.8 g.

COMPLETE PROTEIN

Type of Food	Serving Size	Protein Content
	½ breast	25.7 g.
	1 thigh	15.0 g.
	1 drumstick	12.1 g.
turkey (roasted)	2 pieces (or 3 oz. light meat)	28.0 g.
	4 pieces (or 3 oz. dark meat)	25.5 g.

INCOMPLETE PROTEIN

Bread
white	1 slice	2.4 g.
whole wheat	1 slice	2.4 g.
bran muffin	1	3.1 g.
corn muffin	1	2.8 g.

Cereal
bran flakes	1 cup	3.6 g.
corn grits	1 cup (cooked)	2.9 g.
corn flakes	1 cup (flakes)	2.0 g.
farina	1 cup (cooked)	3.2 g.
oatmeal	1 cup (cooked)	4.8 g.
puffed oats	1 cup	3.0 g.
oven-popped rice	1 cup	1.8 g.
wheat flakes	1 cup	3.1 g.
shredded wheat	1 cup (or 50 small biscuits)	5.0 g.
wheat germ	1 tbsp.	1.8 g.
	1 cup	20.0 g.

Dried Beans
pea (navy) cooked	1 cup	14.8 g.
kidney (cooked)	1 cup	14.4 g.
lima (cooked)	1 cup	12.9 g.
mung	1 cup (sprouts uncooked)	4.0 g.
soybeans (cooked)	1 cup	19.8 g.

Fruits
apricots	3 (raw)	1.1 g.
	10 halves (dried)	2.4 g.
avocado	½ large	2.4 g.

INCOMPLETE PROTEIN

Type of Food	Serving Size	Protein Content
bananas	1	1.5 g.
dates	10	1.8 g.
grapefruit	½ fresh	.5 g.
orange	1	1.3 g.
prunes	1 cup (cooked)	3.4 g.
raisins	1½-oz. package	1.1 g.
strawberries	1 cup fresh	1.0 g.
watermelon	1 (4-in.) wedge	2.0 g.
Pasta		
macaroni	1 cup (cooked)	16.8 g.
noodles (egg)	1 cup (cooked)	6.6 g.
noodles (chow mein)	1 cup	5.9 g.
spaghetti	1 cup (cooked)	6.5 g
Nuts		
almonds	22 nuts (roasted)	5.3 g.
cashews	½ cup	12.0 g.
peanuts	10 large nuts (in shell)	4.7 g.
peanut butter	1 tbsp.	4.0 g.
sunflower seeds	½ cup (hulled)	17.4 g.
walnuts	½ cup (shelled)	7.4 g.
Rice (cooked)		
brown	1 cup	13.9 g.
white	1 cup	12.4 g.
Vegetables		
broccoli (cooked)	1 large stalk	8.7 g.
Brussels sprouts (cooked)	1 cup	6.5 g.
cauliflower (cooked)	1 cup	2.9 g.
corn (cooked)	1 cup	5.3 g.
kale (cooked)	1 cup	5.0 g.
mushrooms	1 cup	1.3 g.
peas (cooked)	1 cup	8.6 g.
potatoes	1 long potato (baked)	4.0 g.

INCOMPLETE PROTEIN

Type of Food	Serving Size	Protein Content
	1 round potato boiled)	2.9 g.
sweet potatoes	1 potato (baked)	2.4 g.
turnips	1 cup	1.3 g.

53. Facts and fallacies about protein

FIRST THE FACTS:

- Children need one-and-a-half to two times more protein per pound of body weight than adults—and babies need two to three times more. (See section 54.)
- Protein helps to develop muscles and keep them healthy.
- You can get more protein per pound with cheaper cuts of meat (because they have less fat).
- The child's body excretes a larger portion of low-quality protein and uses a higher proportion of high-quality protein. (In other words, the better the protein, the less a child needs. The top-quality protein sources—descending from a nearly perfect ''10''—are breast milk, whole egg, whole milk, meat or fish, and rice.)
- The combination of incomplete protein and a complete protein provides more nutritive value than either could alone.

NOW THE FALLACIES:

- *Protein is nonfattening.* This erroneous assumption has put more fat on kids than ice cream! Gram for gram, protein has the same amount of calories as carbohydrates. The truth is:

    1 g. protein   = 4 calories
    1 g. carbohydrate = 4 calories
    1 g. fat   = 9 calories

- *Protein burns up fat.* This is another mistaken conception, and any parent who thinks that three hamburgers without buns are less fattening than one with, will have a child who's going to learn the truth the hard way—round.

- *Protein "builds" muscles*. This is not true if you're thinking of the sort of muscles that bulge the T-shirts of young athletes. Protein does help develop muscles, but "building" them requires exercise.
- *Strenuous activity increases the need for protein*. It might increase the need for calories but not necessarily for protein. A child's protein need depends on size and rate of growth (see table below).

54. How much does my child really need?

There's no one protein requirement for all children. The actual amount of protein needed by any given child depends on a variety of factors, including health, age, height, and weight. To estimate your child's personal daily recommended allowance, use the chart below.

AGE GROUP	1–3	4–6	7–10	11–14	15–18
POUND KEY	0.82	0.68	0.55	0.45	0.40

Example: Your son weighs 100 pounds and is fourteen years old.
His pound key is 0.45.
$0.45 \times 100 = 45$ g.—his daily requirement.

55. How to sneak more into your child's diet

*Camouflaged nutrition is slightly sneaky
—but sensationally successful!*

If you're worried about your child not getting enough protein—and know that asking him to finish his eggs or to eat another piece of fish will get you nowhere—then you're ready for what I call "camouflaged nutrition."

It's not as sneaky as it sounds, and kids love it—provided that you don't announce that you're doing something that's "good for them." As aware of nutrition as children are these days, they're always just a bit suspicious of those three words.

The key to successful camouflaged nutrition is stocking up on high-protein ingredients, such as brewer's yeast, wheat germ, sunflower and sesame seeds (don't use seeds for children under four), powdered milk, eggs, and nuts—and slipping them into the foods your child does eat. (You'll know you've become a master at it when your kids think that they're simply getting extra treats.)

> *Toasting your own sunflower seeds is easy,*
> *fun, and better for your kids.*

Start with breakfast—sprinkle unsalted nuts and seeds on cold cereals. Peanuts and sunflower seeds (a combination that increases in protein when eaten together) can work wonders on little round oats. It's best if you buy the sunflower seeds unroasted and then toast them yourself on a cookie sheet in a 200°–250° oven. Actually, you can toast half the seeds, then put them together with the raw ones in a tightly sealed jar, shake well, let stand at room temperature for a few hours, and all will taste roasted.

You can rev up sandwiches by 6 grams of protein with just one slice of unprocessed cheese, which tastes delicious with tuna fish, luncheon meats, even peanut butter.

Unprocessed cheese can also turn bland rice into a protein-packed treat. Cook rice according to package directions. Then, while the rice is still hot, grate in an ounce or two of cheddar. It melts right in—deliciously. Grated cheddar also works well in salads and on vegetables.

For dinner, try adding nutritional oomph to meals with tofu (soybean curd). This Oriental staple is high in protein and remarkably low in calories, cholesterol, and cost. Because if its mild taste, it works especially well when cut into squares and mixed in soups, salads, or vegetables, absorbing the best flavors from whatever it's combined with.

Bean sprouts—another high-protein, low-calorie food—work well mixed in tuna salad. And if your kids like Chinese-style food, you can sauté mung-bean sprouts in sesame oil with garlic, a pinch of ginger, tamari, and vegetables—they'll think they're eating out!

A cup of nonfat dry milk has 43 grams of protein; it can be added, without your child's knowing it, to breads and cakes, as well as hot cereals and soups. Yogurt is a fine fortifier, too. (See section 82 for recipes.)

Wheat germ adds both flavor and nutrients to meat loaves, cereals, soups, and breads. It can also be used as a topping for cooked vegetables.

One of the easiest ways to get your child to like wheat germ is with Miss Winne's Wonderful Banana Pops. The kids can make these themselves:

1. Cut one firm banana in half crosswise.
2. Insert a popsickle stick through the cut side of each half.
3. Roll each half in milk—then roll the milked half in wheat germ.
4. Place on waxed paper in freezer.

They should be frozen delicious in about an hour.

And for a real protein lift that can keep kids who are on the go really going, I recommend my Powerhouse Plus.

POWERHOUSE PLUS

8 oz. apple juice (unsweetened)
½ small banana
3 or 4 ripe strawberries
3 or 4 ice cubes
2 tbsp. protein powder (milk and egg protein powder works best)

2 tbsp. lecithin granules
1 tbsp. yeast (if protein powder already contains yeast, this can be omitted)

1. Pour the juice into the blender first, and keeping the blender on low, add the fruit.
2. When blended, add the ice cubes, then the protein powder, lecithin granules, and yeast.
3. Turn blender to high until mixture looks deliciously smooth.

By the way, this is great for parents on the go, too. This mixture can be frozen and served as power popsicles.

56. Caring about carbohydrates

Carbohydrates have had bad press. Most people think of them as villains, but just because some are, doesn't mean they all are. In moderation, carbohydrates are indispensable to a child's metabolic process. Their chief function is to provide a child with energy and to assist in the digestion and assimilation of all the foods he eats. (Unrefined products supply fiber.)

Carbohydrates break down inside cells to release energy. In fact, the primary source of the brain's energy is the sugar glucose, which comes mainly from starch in the diet. But if the energy is not needed, the carbohydrates are stored in the liver as glycogen for later use. Unfortunately, since there's a limit to what the liver can handle, the excess is converted into body fat. The more excess, the more fat. And as if this weren't trouble enough, the excess can also cause a vitamin B deficiency because the child's B vitamins will be called from other metabolic needs to burn up the unnecessary carbohydrates.

HOW MUCH IS ENOUGH?

One gram of carbohydrate daily for each three pounds of your child's body weight.

HOW TO TELL THE GOOD GUYS FROM THE BAD GUYS

THE GOOD GUYS
Whole grains—wheat, rye, barley
Whole-grain cereals
Whole-grain breads
Brown rice
Vegetables
Fresh vegetable juices
Fresh fruit juices
Fruits

THE OKAY GUYS
Natural brown sugar
Honey
Unsulfured molasses
Maple sugar
Dried fruit
Carob powder

THE BAD GUYS

Refined white sugar

Potato chips

Snack pies, cakes, and cookies

Carbonated soft drinks

Chocolate candy bars

Chewing gum

Sugared breakfast cereal

57. The importance of fats

In a child's diet, fats are as necessary as protein or carbohydrates—but not in the same amounts. They offer twice as many calories per gram as proteins or carbohydrates, which is why only 25 percent of a child's daily calories needs to come from fats.

HOW THEY HELP YOUR CHILD

- Aid in hormone development.
- Ensure proper structure of all cells—especially those essential for memory and digestion.
- Promote healthy blood vessels.
- Assist in proper transmission of nerve-to-muscle impulses.
- Assist in controlling the functions of key glands and important chemical reactions necessary to enable enzymes to work.
- Provide the necessary elements for absorption of oil-soluble vitamins—such as vitamins A, D, E, and K—and other nutrients.
- Make foods more palatable.

58. Knowing the fats

Though all fats contain the same chemical elements of glycerol and fatty acids, they're not persent in the same order or amounts in each. (The three essential fatty acids, which the body cannot produce, are linoleic, arachidonic, and linolenic; these are known as vitamin F.) (See section 22.)

Saturated fat is the type that's usually solid when at room temperature. This is found in meats (coconut, too) and can increase the amount of cholesterol in the blood. Cholesterol, which is essential in the skin for converting the sun's ultraviolet rays to vitamin D, is necessary in the liver for creating bile acids, and is a prime supplier of cortisone and sex hormones, can cling to the inner walls of blood vessels, making it difficult for the blood to pass.

Unsaturated fat (monounsaturated or polyunsaturated) is usually liquid and comes primarily from vegetable sources. Unsaturated fats do not raise cholesterol levels, and polyunsaturated fats actually lower them!

FOODS FOR THOUGHT

- Processed luncheon meats, such as hot dogs, Spam, bacon, and bologna, are high in saturated fat and offer poor compensation in protein, vitamins, and minerals.
- Fish fat is both polyunsaturated *and* saturated, but there are *more* polyunsaturates, especially in mackerel and halibut. Fish canned in cottonseed oil, though not peanut or olive oil, is also higher in polyunsaturated fat.
- Eggs, which do contain saturated fat, also contain lecithin, which *aids in the assimilation of fat*. In fact, eggs can raise the blood level of HDL, high-density lipoproteins whose detergent action can actually break up cholesterol. (Though the American Heart Association still deems eggs a cholesterol hazard, recent research from the National Research Council disputes this.)

If you are concerned about the amount of cholesterol your child is getting from convenience foods, be sure to check the labels.

59. Calorie requirements from infancy to adolescence

Before putting your child on a diet or assuming that he or she is eating too much or too little, it's important to know what his calorie needs really are. The following chart should help.

CALORIE NEEDS FOR KIDS

Age (Years)	Approximate Weight (lbs.)	Approximate Calories	To Find Your Own Child's Calorie Needs Multiply Weight by
1–3	28	1,300	46
3–6	44	1,800	41
7–10	66	2,400	36
(M) 11–14	97	2,800	29
15–18	134	3,000	22½
(F) 11–14	97	2,400	25
15–18	119	2,100	18

60. Yea, for Yeast!

> *If Nature gave Academy Awards for vitamins, yeast would definitely win an Oscar.*

Not only is one tablespoon an excellent source of protein (36 percent) and a superior source of B-complex vitamins, it is a veritable treasure trove of minerals, trace minerals, and amino acids—and one of the richest suppliers of organic iron.

It is also the *best* nutritional source of chromium, which occurs in brewer's yeast as an organic compound known as GTF (Glucose Tolerance Factor). GTF is essential for the production of insulin, necessary for managing the body's major fuel, glucose.

Easily stirred into soups, shakes, juices, or foods, it's probably the simplest way to sneakily, and *pleasantly,* enrich your child's diet.

Here's what I call The Dynamite Lunchbox Special:

> Blend some brewer's yeast with peanut butter (the nutlike flavors are very compatible). Make a sandwich with a little sliced banana and this home-fortified peanut butter, and your child should come through a long school afternoon with energy to spare.

There are various sources of yeast, and they're all good guys except one—*live baker's yeast! Avoid it!* The live yeast cells can deplete B vitamins and rob your child of even more vitamins. What you should look for are nutritional yeasts. In these the live cells have been heat-killed to prevent any sort of depletion.

Brewer's yeast (made from hops, a by-product of beer), often called nutritional yeast.

Torula yeast (grown on wood pulp used in the manufacture of paper or from blackstrap molasses), which is sometimes added to commercial baby foods as a flavor enhancer.

Whey, a by-product of milk and cheese, made famous by Little Miss Muffit, and possibly the best-tasting and most potent of the lot.

Liquid yeast, which comes from Switzerland and Germany, and is fed on herbs, honey malt, and oranges or grapefruit.

Most yeast that is purchased as a food supplement has calcium already added to it (read the label). If not, you'll have to make sure your child is getting extra calcium because yeast, like other protein foods, is high in phosphorus, which can take calcium out of the body.

61. Any questions about chapter IV?

I've put my son on a high-protein diet, eliminated junk foods and all fats, but he hasn't lost much weight. Why is this?

There could be a number of reasons. Feeding a child lots of protein does not mean that you're giving him fewer calories. And if the protein you're giving him includes steaks, pork chops, cheeses, and eggs, he's getting plenty of fat nonetheless. And if he's eating larger amounts of meat, he's consuming a great number of calories. Balancing his diet and checking calorie counts is more sensible and more effective. (See section 59.)

You're right for eliminating junk foods; but bear in mind that luncheon meats, such as bologna, processed ham spreads, and hot dogs (which many parents unwittingly believe are good protein sources), contain hidden carbohydrates and fats that far outweigh the value of their protein. Also, make sure your son is exercising. If he's downing big steaks and sitting around watching TV, he's not going to lose much weight.

I'm inclined to doubt that his problem is metabolic. But if you balance his meals and are sure he's not secretly snacking, and he still doesn't lose weight, it would be advisable to check with a nutritionally oriented doctor.

My toddler refuses to drink water. Milk and juice, yes, but never plain water. Is it necessary?

It's good for him but not necessary if he's getting enough liquids in one form or another daily. Four to six glasses of liquid is sufficient for a toddler. But I would suggest increasing the fruits in his diet. And try gradually diluting one glass of juice a day, in an effort to get him acquainted with plain water.

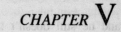

CHAPTER V

Your Child's Vitamin Needs

62. Why parents must be detectives

Because many vitamin-deficiency symptoms could also be symptoms of other diseases, it's important for you to be aware of what your child *is* or *is not* eating and to be able to supply this information to a doctor.

> *It's difficult for even the best doctor to make the right diagnosis without the right facts.*

For example, a child with dermatitis might simply be told not to wear wool or other irritating fabrics if the parent hasn't informed the doctor that the child consumes mostly carbohydrates, doesn't drink milk, and rarely eats eggs or vegetables, which would indicate a possible biotin deficiency. Or a doctor might assume that your child's bright red tongue is a reaction to a medication he's taking because you haven't mentioned the child's avoidance of nutritious vitamin-B-rich foods. No one can come up with the right solution with the wrong clues.

63. Causes of vitamin deficiencies in children

You can easily be misled into thinking that because your child is the proper weight—or even overweight—he couldn't possibly have a vitamin deficiency. But this isn't so. What you have to realize is that nourishment is *not* determined by the number of calories consumed. In fact, junk foods—especially those high in refined white sugar and those that are processed, emulsified, and dye-colored—need B-complex vitamins for digestion and metabolization. And if your child isn't getting enough of these B vitamins in his daily food, his body will take those needed for other essential uses, and deficiency and illness will occur.

OTHER CAUSES OF CHILDREN'S VITAMIN DEFICIENCIES

- An infant who spits up feedings repeatedly tends to have an inadequate food intake and therefore an inadequate vitamin intake.
- During illness or rapid-growth spurts, a child's formerly adequate diet can become insufficient in essential nutrients.
- An intestinal disease or organ malfunction that causes poor vitamin absorption.
- An insufficient amount of dietary fat for proper absorption of oil-soluble vitamins.

64. Deficiency diseases, symptoms, and warning signals

Deficiencies don't happen overnight, and it's far better to spot one coming than to wait until the nutrient itself is too far gone. (A B_{12} deficiency may take five years to appear *after* the body has been depleted). What follows is a list of known deficiency diseases, the nutrient whose deficiency can cause them, and the symptoms of each disease. After this list I describe certain warning signals to watch for and indicate the nutrient whose deficiency may explain them.

Disease	Deficiency	Symptoms
Beriberi	Vitamin B_1 (Thiamine)	Muscular atrophy and nerve weakness causing paralysis of the legs
Hypoprothrom-binemia	Vitamin K	Poor blood clotting
Hypothyroid-ism	Iodine	Enlargement of thyroid gland, slowing mental reactions and often causing obesity
Iron-deficiency Anemia	Iron	Fatigue, pale skin

Disease	Deficiency	Symptoms
Night Blindness	Vitamin A	Inability to see under twilight or dusk conditions
Pellagra	Niacin	Redness like sunburn, burning and itching on parts of exposed skin, especially when rubbed; weakness and loss of appetite
Pernicious Anemia	Vitamin B_{12}	Gastrointestinal difficulties and numbness or other sensory disturbance in the limbs
Rickets	Vitamin D	Malformed bones and teeth
Scurvy	Vitamin C	Bleeding gums, joint pains, extreme overall weakness
Tetany	Vitamin D	Violent muscular spasm and cramps, sometimes convulsions
Xerophthalmia	Vitamin A	Thickened mucous membranes around the eyes, impairing vision
Xerosis	Vitamin A	Eyeball loses luster and becomes dry and inflamed

Warning Signals	*Possible Deficiency Developing*
Impaired night vision, diarrhea, intestinal infection; rough, dry skin; frequent sties in the eye; multiple skin blemishes.	Vitamin A
Loss of appetite, decreased mental alertness, poor memory, irritability, lack of energy.	Vitamin B_1 (Thiamine)
Cracks at the corner of the mouth; sore, red tongue;	Vitamin B_2 (Riboflavin)

Warning Signals	*Possible Deficiency Developing*
gritty feeling behind the lids; scaly skin around the nose, mouth, forehead, and ears; sensitivity to light.	
Low blood sugar, cracks around the mouth, muscle twitching, irritability, dermatitis near eyes, numbness and cramps in limbs; slow learning, frequent urination.	Vitamin B_6 (Pyridoxine)
Soreness in arms and legs, pins-and-needles feeling in limbs, poor memory, stammering, feeling of soreness in mouth, difficulties in walking, poor reflexes.	Vitamin B_{12}
Fatigue, nausea, depression, dry skin, muscular pains, insomnia.	Biotin
Blocked kidney tubes, stomach ulcers.	Choline
Red tongue, diarrhea, intestinal disturbances, low hematocrit.	Folic Acid (Folacin)
Eczema, constipation.	Inositol
Appetite loss, bad breath, canker sores, sore gums, headaches, vertigo, skin and gastrointestinal lesions.	Niacin
Fatigue, sleep disturbances, burning feet, nausea. (Deficiencies are rare, though, because pantothenic acid is found in most foods.)	Pantothenic Acid
Bruising easily, bleeding gums, nosebleeds, painful joints, slow healing of wounds.	Vitamin C

Warning Signals	*Possible Deficiency Developing*
Softening of the skull, enlargements of joints, fragile bones, bowed legs.	Vitamin D
Possible anemia in premature or low birth-weight infants.	Vitamin E
Brittle hair, dandruff, dry skin, brittle nails.	Vitamin F
Irritability, cramps, joint pains, tooth decay	Calcium
Slow learning ability, obesity, poor memory.	Iodine
Pale skin, fatigue.	Iron
Muscle twitchiness, mental disorientation.	Magnesium
Slow growth, unhealthy teeth.	Phosphorus
Nervousness, insomnia, constipation, fatigue, acne.	Potassium
Fatigue, poor growth, lusterless hair, brittle nails, poor appetite.	Protein
Intestinal gas, weight loss. (Rare because of the high salt content in foods children eat.)	Sodium
White spots on nails, poor attention, fatigue, high susceptibility to infection.	Zinc

65. Tests for deficiencies

If you suspect that your child is deficient in any nutrient, my advice is that you consult a nutritionally oriented doctor to confirm your suspicion before putting the child on a full-scale supplement regimen. If you don't know of any in your area, the International Academy of Preventive Medicine, 10409 Town & Country Way, Suite 200, Houston, Texas 77024, offers listings on request. (See section 171 for additional listings.)

To test your child for a mineral deficiency (or surplus), you need only a tablespoon or two of his hair to send to a lab for analysis. Some laboratories will send results only to doctors, but others will send them to individuals. It's best to query the lab first. (You can try the Soil and Health Foundation of Emmaus, Pennsylvania 18049; or Parmae Laboratories, Inc., P.O. Box 35227, Dallas, Texas 75235; or Hartley Research Labs, 1495 West Street, Provo, Utah 84601.)

If you would just like to determine whether your child is getting enough vitamin C, there is a simple, fairly accurate test that you can do yourself.

VITAMIN C TEST

Materials:

10 drops	5 percent solution of aqueous silver nitrate (which can be purchased at almost any drugstore without prescription)
10 drops	child's urine
2	paper cups
1	medicine dropper

Procedure:

Put 10 drops of the aqueous silver nitrate solution in a paper cup. Collect a sample of your child's urine in the other cup, then add ten drops to the aqueous silver nitrate. Let this stand two minutes. The solution will change color—from white to gray to charcoal—depending on the amount of vitamin C being excreted.

The darker the solution, the more vitamin C being excreted, which means the less your child needs. If the solution stays quite light, very little C is being excreted (which means the child needs and is using all he has).

If this is the case, you should increase the child's intake of citrus fruits and leafy greens. (Strawberries are high in C and delicious with cold breakfast cereals; they're great with yogurt for dessert, too.)

Retest in about a week. If there's no improvement, you might want to consider a chewable vitamin C supplement (with bioflavonoids and *no* added sugar), 50–100 mg. once or twice a day, depending on your child's age. (See section 17, "Daily Minimum for Optimum Health.")

Note: Many drugs, illnesses, and foods can also alter urine color. This should be taken into consideration when you test.

66. Hypervitaminosis—how to spot it

It is equally as important to recognize an oversupply of a vitamin as it is to recognize a deficiency; and because infants and children are more susceptible to the adverse effects of overdosage, it's even more so. Too often parents think that if a little of one vitamin is good for a child, a lot will be better; but this is not the case—especially with the following:

Nutrient	*Some Symptoms of Overconsumption*
Vitamin A	mouth ulcers, anemia, nausea, irritability, blurred vision, dry skin, hair loss, sore lips, vomiting, enlargement of the liver, a buildup of pressure within the head that mimics a brain tumor, headaches, bone pain, abdominal pain, brittle nails.
Vitamin C	diarrhea, skin rashes, burning sensation during urination
Vitamin D	nausea, vomiting, appetite loss, weight loss, headaches, calcification of soft tissues, increased frequency of urination, diarrhea, dizziness, muscle weakness (hypercalcemia)
Niacin	jaundice, flushing of the skin (not dangerous but uncomfortable), throbbing in the head, cramps

If your child is taking any of these supplements and the symptoms of overconsumption develop, reduce the dosage and the symptoms should disappear. If they don't, the condition is being caused by other factors and should be brought to the attention of a physician.

67. Hypervitaminosis—how to avoid it

• *Read vitamin labels.* If you've been instructed to give your child a vitamin A supplement, make sure you're not double-dosing by giving him a multivitamin that also contains A. Since vitamins and minerals come in different strengths, check to see that you're not getting more than you asked for.

- *Try the five-day week*. To prevent buildup, give your child supplements only five days a week.
- *Try natural foods before supplements*. (One cup of diced cooked carrots contain 15,230 IU of vitamin A.)

68. How and when to administer vitamins to children

> *Vitamin drops in baby's bottle might not get to baby.*

Doctors often prescribe supplementary vitamins in drop form for infants when they're about two weeks of age. Although parents can add these to the formula, I don't advise it. The liquid may adhere with the milk to the side of the bottle. If the child doesn't finish his bottle, he won't get all the vitamins, and vitamins A, C, and D are particularly important at this time.

- Vitamins can be measured more accurately and administered more efficiently by being dropped directly onto the infant's tongue. (Babies usually like the taste, believe it or not.)

or

- Mix vitamins with a *small* quantity of juice (or water) if you're fairly certain that the child will finish it.

or

- Once the child starts on solid foods, you can put the vitamins on the feeding spoon and just slip them in his mouth.

For older children who have to have supplements and can't swallow pills:

- Try chewable vitamins, but check the label because many contain unnecessary amounts of sugar. (You might be better off buying a regular tablet, crushing it, and mixing it with some honey and apple sauce.)
- Use liquid preparations that mix easily with juices and food.

- Pierce vitamin A or E capsules with a pin, and then squeeze the vitamin onto a spoon and mix with a small amount of honey.

VITAMINS WORK BEST WHEN TAKEN WITH FOOD!

69. What to look for when buying vitamins for children

Natural vitamins! Although chemically the same as synthetic vitamins, natural vitamins have been found to cause fewer gastrointestinal upsets in children. And, more important, natural vitamins will not cause the toxic reactions that can occur with synthetic vitamins when taken in higher than usual doses. Noted allergist Dr. Theron G. Randolph explains it this way:

> A synthetically derived substance may cause a reaction in a chemically susceptible person when the same material of natural origin is tolerated, despite the two substances having identical chemical structures.

All vitamins are "organic," but they're not all "natural."

Be forewarned that the difference between "inorganic" and "organic" is *not* the same as that between "synthetic" and "natural."

- All vitamins are *organic* (which simply means they contain carbon). Don't be fooled into thinking you're buying natural vitamins just because the word "organic" is on the label. *Read carefully.* A new truth-in-labeling law for vitamins has recently gone into effect. This means that *all* ingredients in the formula, not just the vitamins and minerals, but the fillers, binders, diluents, lubricants, colors, flavors, coating materials, and drying agents will be listed on the label in descending order. This means the first ingredient (the majority by weight in the tablet, capsule, or liquid) is listed first, and so on down the line.
- Most minerals, on the other hand, are inorganic (which means they don't contain carbon). Some organic excep-

tions are the irons—ferrous gluconate, ferrous peptonate, and ferrous citrate. (Ferrous sulfate, however, is an inorganic iron.)

- When buying mineral supplements, look for those that are chelated (pronounced *key-lated*). These are assimilated faster and are therefore more effective.
- Store all vitamins away from light and heat and moisture.
- Remove cotton that comes in vitamin bottles.
- Date vitamins (if the date isn't on the label) and discard open bottles after a year. (Unopened bottles can be kept for two years.)
- *Keep all vitamins out of the reach of children.*

70. Any questions about chapter V?

Is there any sugar in children's vitamins?

Is there! It's the first ingredient in virtually *all* vitamins for kids, and in some it's the second and third as well! I can't emphasize enough the importance of reading labels. Many children's vitamins also contain artificial colors and flavorings, salt, and other additives. When you consider that sugar, additives, and artificial colors have been found to influence hyperactivity and other behavioral disorders in children (see section 103), you realize how essential it is to read the manufacturer's small print—even on vitamins.

Here are a few big offenders:

TRI-VI-SOL CHEWABLE TABLETS
First ingredient (the majority) sugar (great for dental cavities . . . second ingredient glucose (more sugar!) . . . artificial color and flavor . . . salt listed as seventh ingredient . . . sodium ascorbate listed as tenth ingredient (more sodium).

POLY-VI-SOL WITH IRON DROPS
First ingredient is glycerin . . . third ingredient is polysorbate 80, a homogenizer or solubilizer also used as a laundry detergent.

VI-DAYLIN CHEWABLE VITAMINS
First ingredient is sucrose (sugar) . . . second ingredient is dextrin (another sugar-type carbohydrate) . . . artificial flavor ("artificial cherry") and artificial color.

VI-DAYLIN HOMOGENIZED LIQUID MULTIVITAMIN
First ingredient glucose . . . second ingredient sucrose
. . . third ingredient polysorbate 80.

ACACIA
Cysteine HCL as a stabilizer . . . benzoic acid as a
preservative.

ONE-A-DAY VITAMINS PLUS MINERALS
Dicalcium phosphate—a filler, first ingredient . . .
cellulose—a filler, third ingredient . . . starch—a filler,
sixth ingredient . . . gelatin . . . artificial color . . .
propylene glycol (which is also used as an antifreeze)
. . . hydroxypropylmethylcellulose . . . magnesium stearate . . . polyvinylpyrrolidone . . . silica . . . ethyl
cellulose . . . polysorbate 80 . . . artificial flavor.

CHOCKS CHEWABLE MULTIVITAMIN
First ingredient sucrose . . . third ingredient cellulose
. . . fourth ingredient stearic acid . . . fifth ingredient
dextrin (a carbohydrate) . . . magnesium stearate . . .
artificial colors . . . glycerides of stearic acid and palmitic
acids.

FLINTSTONE'S CHILDREN'S CHEWABLE VITAMINS
The container boasts, "Many doctors recommend." I'm
sure they haven't read the label, because the ingredients
are sodium, ascorbate, stearic acid, gelatin, dextrin, artificial flavors, artificial colors.

My advice is: Buy a brand that states on the label, "No
sugar, no starch, no artificial flavors or colors or artificial
preservatives." Your kids get too much of them already.

CHAPTER VI

Vitamin Facts Parents Are the Last to Know

71. Be cautious when you mix kids and vitamins

There's no doubt that kids thrive on the right vitamins, but there are times and circumstances when some of them are *not* recommended. Medicines, a variety of metabolic conditions—even vitamins themselves—can be affected by certain vitamins (and vice versa) both positively and negatively.

For this reason I advise you to look over the following list carefully. Your children deserve nothing but the best from vitamins—and by knowing these facts you can feel confident that is just what they're getting.

- Children being treated for acne or other dermatological conditions with medications containing large doses of vitamin A can develop chronic hypervitaminosis A.
- Large intakes of sugar, cola, and chocolate deplete your child of vitamin B_1 (thiamine).
- Too much vitamin B_1 can affect thyroid and insulin production.
- Symptoms of a vitamin B_{12} deficiency may take as long as five years to appear *after* the child's body has been depleted.
- Antacids (such as Tums, Rolaids, Maalox) when used too often can deplete a child's system of phosphate and lead to muscle weakness.
- Poor skin conditions can be worsened with iodine. (Check label of vitamin-mineral supplement the child is taking—and have the child avoid iodized salt.)
- An iron supplement (ferrous sulfate or ferrous chloride) will have inhibited absorption if taken with milk.

- Supplementary vitamin D and iron are required by breast-fed infants and those receiving unfortified cow's milk.
- A child taking megadoses of vitamin C can deplete needed stores of vitamin B_{12} and folic acid.
- Too much salt in the child's diet can cause potassium loss.
- Vitamin B_6 should not be taken by anyone under L-dopa treatment (rarely used for children under 17.)
- Taking only one B vitamin over a prolonged period of time can significantly deplete the others.
- An excess of stored vitamin D, which promotes absorption of calcium, can cause hypercalcemia (too much calcium in the blood).
- If your child is diabetic and taking vitamin C, it might be necessary to *lower* the dosage of medication (check with the doctor).
- Raw egg whites can deactivate your child's biotin supply.
- Large amounts of vitamin C can reverse the anticoagulant activity of blood-thinning medications.
- An excessive intake of leafy vegetables—especially spinach, cauliflower, Brussels sprouts, and potatoes—can also reverse the anticoagulant activity of blood-thinning medications. (The high vitamin C and K content of these foods decreases the drug's activity.)
- To promote absorption, children being treated for ringworm or other fungus infections with griseofulvin, (Fulvicin, ® Grifulvin® V, Grisactin®) should increase their fat intake while on the medication.
- Large doses of choline, taken over an extended period of time, can produce a deficiency of vitamin B_6.
- Children with heart disorders should have their vitamin D dosages prescribed by a physician.
- Vitamin E should be given cautiously to any child with an overactive thyroid, diabetes, high blood pressure, or rheumatic heart. (A child with any of these conditions could be started on a very low dosage, which can gradually be increased.)
- Premature infants on restricted diets may need vitamin E supplementations.
- Vitamin E has enabled diabetics to reduce their insulin levels. (Check with your child's physician.)

- A child with rheumatic fever (or rheumatic heart) has an imbalance between the two sides of the heart, and large vitamin E doses can increase the imbalance and worsen the condition. (Consult the child's doctor before using supplements.)
- Vitamin E can elevate blood pressure in hypertensive children, but if the supplementation is started with a low dosage and increased very slowly, there will be an eventual lowering of the pressure because of the vitamin's diuretic properties.
- A child with a history of convulsive disorders should not be given large doses of folic acid for any extended period of time.
- An oversupply of folic acid can mask symptoms of pernicious anemia.
- Folic acid and PABA can inhibit the effectiveness of sulfonamides, such as Gantricin.
- A child who eats large amounts of meat, eggs, cheese, and milk needs extra vitamin B_6.
- Carrots and liver won't give an effective amount of vitamin A to a child with a zinc deficiency.
- When adding zinc to a diet, be sure there's sufficient vitamin A.
- Vitamin C, taken *with* meals, makes dietary iron more readily available to a child. (This is especially important for vegatarian children. As a general rule, fiber inhibits iron absorption.)
- Niacin should be given cautiously to children with diabetes, glaucoma, ulcer, or liver problems.
- Iron-deficiency anemia is the most prevalent nutritional deficiency in infants.
- Iron should not be taken by any child with sickle-cell anemia, hemochromatosis, or thalassemia.
- Ferrous sulfate iron supplements can decrease a child's vitamin E.
- A child's iron absorption can be inhibited by large intakes of chocolate, cola, and other beverages containing caffeine.
- Too much manganese can reduce utilization of iron.
- Excessive doses of iron-fortified vitamins or over-the-counter medicinal iron formulas can cause iron poisoning in children.

- If a child's diet is high in fat, it can increase phosphorus absorption and lower calcium levels.
- If your child is taking medication for an underactive thyroid gland, be aware that kelp can affect that gland. If you've added kelp to the child's diet, he might need *less* prescription medicine.
- Large amounts of raw cabbage can cause an iodine deficiency and lower thyroid production in children with existing low-iodine intakes.
- An inositol shortage can occur in a child who consumes large amounts of cola, chocolate, and other products containing caffeine.
- Inform the doctor if your child is taking supplementary C because vitamin C can alter results of lab tests.
- Popcorn is a good source of fiber in a child's diet (though not for children under four).
- If you give your child tryptophan as a natural relaxant, do not have him take it with milk or other protein—use juice or water.
- For optimum absorption of a vitamin A supplement, the child should not engage in strenuous physical activity for at least two hours.
- Extra calcium can relieve a child's muscle cramps after exercise.
- Mineral oil robs your child of vitamins A, D, E, and K.

72. Any questions about chapter VI?

Are there any vitamins that can release more iron from natural foods?

Vitamin C—but your child must take it *with* the meal. The truth about iron is that even though it is present in many foods, that's no guarantee that the child will be able to absorb it. The iron in meats, fish, and poultry is usually easily absorbed, but the iron in vegetables and beans, for instance, is not. Vegetarian children especially should take vitamin C with their meals and avoid drinking tea or eating high-fiber foods at that time, since both can inhibit iron absorption.

I've heard that vitamins are being used in the treatment of schizophrenic children. What vitamins are these?

There are a variety of vitamin treatments for schizophrenic children now being tested. Most include the B vitamins—primarily vitamins B_1, B_3, B_6, and B_{12}. According to the *Journal of Orthomolecular Psychiatry,* studies done by Dr. Stanley Krippner and Stewart Fisher, as well as recent ones by Dr. Bernard Rimland, Dr. E. Calloway, and Dr. Pierre Dryfus, have proved hearteningly successful.

Is there any danger of toxicity from consuming large amounts of vegetables containing vitamin A?

No. Unlike preformed vitamin A, which comes from animal sources, carotenoids—which are found in vegetable sources—are converted to vitamin A in the intestine, and there is no danger of their being toxic.

Are there any vitamins that have been able to help autistic children?

Dr. Bernard Rimland of San Diego has found that vitamin B_6 (400–500 mg.) daily has benefited autistic children.

Are some children more prone than others to vitamin deficiencies?

Yes. Any child who gets one-quarter or more of his daily calories from nutritionally deficient foods, such as refined carbohydrates, sugary beverages, candies, and other snacks, is more likely to be deficient in adequate nutrients.

Part Two

BRINGING UP
BABY—RIGHT!

CHAPTER VII

Formula vs. Breast-feeding

73. The pros and cons

> *Breast-feeding is strongly recommended for full-term infants, except in the instances where specific contraindications exist.*
>
> —AMERICAN ACADEMY OF PEDIATRICS
> COMMITTEE ON NUTRITION

> *Recent findings of organochlorine insecticides such as DDT, PCBs, and other environmental pollutants in breast milk have raised questions which have not as yet been resolved in regard to the safety of breast-feeding by all mothers.*
> —AMERICAN ACADEMY OF PEDIATRICS
> COMMITTEE ON NUTRITION

BREAST MILK

Pro
- Regarded as the most desirable source of nutrients for the very young infant.
- Supplies nutrients that are not available in any other form.
- Well tolerated by infant; low incidence of allergic response.
- Protects child by providing it with antibodies from the mother.
- Psychologically beneficial to mother and baby.

- Milk produced by the mother of a premature infant is uniquely suited to that infant's nutritional requirements (has more protein than mature milk).
- Continually adapts to the baby's changing needs. (It's high in protein soon after birth to meet the infant's tremendous growth requirement; later, protein decreases and more carbohydrates are formed to fill increasing energy demands.)
- Babies are well nourished on fewer total ounces because nutritional needs are met by proper amount of minerals. Cow-milk formulas contain surplus minerals that must be excreted in extra water.
- Breast-fed babies have fewer colds, allergies, rashes, and are rarely constipated.
- The calcium of human milk is used more efficiently than is that of cow's milk.
- Human milk is an excellent source of tryptophan.
- Prevents infant from being exposed to emulsifiers, additives such as carrageenan, sodium citrate, thickening agents, and pH adjusters that are found in formulas but not in human milk.
- Prevents overfeeding, which can contribute to subsequent obesity because of overproduction of fat cells.

Con

- The amount of iron in human milk is low.
- The amount of B_6 in human milk is low.
- If the mother's diet is insufficient in nutrients, her breast milk will also be insufficient.
- Pollutants in mother's milk will be passed on to baby.

FORMULA MILK

Pro

- Can serve as the sole source of nutrients for a newborn.
- Providing adequate caloric intake for low-birth-weight infants can be facilitated by feeding formulas of caloric density greater than that of human milk.
- The breast-fed baby is more susceptible than the formula-fed baby to hemorrhage caused by lack of vitamin K.
- If mother is taking medication, drugs excreted can alter

milk composition and adversely affect the infant. (See section 74.)
- Human milk contains more DDT than cow's milk.
- Formula variations provide the opportunity to select a product that satisfies the special nutritional requirements of a particular infant.
- Breast milk cannot be given to a child born with PKU (phenylketonuria).
- Bottle-fed babies demonstrate a greater gain in weight and length than breast-fed infants.

Con
- Many infant formulas contain additives, such as carrageenan—a milk-stabilizing agent that is suspected of causing gastrointestinal illnesses—and coconut oil (said to be a contributing factor to hardening of the arteries).
- Constipation is more likely in bottle-fed babies.
- Infants are not supplied the immunities provided by breast milk.

74. You have to be twice as careful when you're feeding two

If you are a nursing mother, you're the sole source of your child's food supply, and your milk is only as rich in nutrients as those you can provide.

Your daily diet should include:

Milk—a quart a day (low-fat, fat-free, whole, evaporated, or skimmed) in any form. And extra fluids.

Meat, fish, poultry, eggs—at least one serving a day. (Liver once a week gives a nutritional boost.)

Fruits and vegetables—several servings daily, and they should include plenty of leafy dark-green vegetables and fresh vitamin-C-rich fruits.

Whole-grain cereals and breads—three servings to provide ample B vitamins.

A multivitamin-mineral supplement that provides enough vitamin D to allow you to properly use the calcium in your diet.

Consult your doctor about any medications you're taking. Many drugs can enter breast milk—and what's good for you is not necessarily good for your child.

DRUGS THAT MAY HARM A NURSING BABY

Anthroquinone laxatives
Atropine
Barbiturates (large doses)
Bishydroxycoumarin
Chloramphenicol
Corticosteroids
Cyclophosphamide
Diazepam
Ergot alkaloids
Estrogens
Isoniazid
Lithium carbonate
Meprobamate
Methotrexate
Metronidazole

Nalidixic acid
Oral contraceptives
Penicillin G
Phenytoin
Potassium iodide
Predinisone
Primidone
Reserpine
Streptomycin
Sulfisoxazole
Tetracycline
Thiazides
Thiouracil
Warfarin

75. Some facts about formulas

Between your child's birth and first birthday his rate of growth is phenomenal, faster than at any other time. Babies usually double their birth-weight by six months and triple it in a year, which is why good nutrition during this stage is vital.

WHAT YOU SHOULD KNOW

- A proper infant formula should contain all the essential nutrients in adequate *but not excessive* amounts; have a sensible distribution of calories derived from easily digestible protein, carbohydrate, and fat sources.
- Evaporated milk and unmodified cow's milk fail to meet current standards for ascorbic acid, vitamin E, and essential fatty acids.
- A formula with too much lactose can cause diarrhea and result in dehydration.
- Infants who are on a skim milk formula over an extended period of time can deplete stores of fat needed for coping with illness.
- Goat's milk formulas are deficient in folic acid. (Infants whose diets are solely goat's milk require about 50 mcg. folic acid as a supplement.)

- Commercial iron-fortified formulas provide adequate iron for infants. Unnecessary supplementation can cause poor absorption of vitamin E and engender hemolytic anemia in premature babies.
- Formulas can be altered by manufacturers because of market availability of ingredients. (Ross modified the fat source in Similac by adding soy oil to their combination of corn and coconut oils because of the rising cost and unavailability of corn oil.)
- If an accurate knowledge of ingredients in your child's formula is important, write to the manufacturer. Changes are often made before new labels are printed, and the information on the product can be incorrect!

76. Special formulas for special situations

LACTOSE INTOLERANCE

Lactose (known as milk sugar) is the most common carbohydrate source in formulas because it is more easily digested than starch. But some infants, especially premature ones, have a lactose intolerance that becomes evident in the first weeks after birth with the occurrence of abdominal distention, diarrhea, and cramps, and must be put on formulas containing alternate carbohydrate sources.

LACTOSE-FREE FORMULAS

Name (manufacturer)	*Carbohydrate source*
Isomil (Ross)	sucrose, corn syrup
i-Soyalac (Loma Linda)	sucrose
Meat Base Formula (Gerber)	sucrose, modified tapioca, starch
Mull-Soy (Syntex)	sucrose, inverted sucrose
Neo-Mull-Soy (Syntex)	sucrose
Nursoy (Wyeth)	sucrose, corn syrup
Nutramigen (Mead Johnson)	sucrose, arrowroot
Pro-Sobee (Mead Johnson)	sucrose, corn syrup, solids
Soyalac (Loma Linda)	sucrose, dextrose, maltose, dextrins

(There is now a lactase liquid and tablet for children with lactose intolerance. See section 83.)

PKU (PHENYLKETONURIA)

This hereditary disease, which can cause mental retardation unless detected and treated early, is caused by the lack of an enzyme needed to convert phenylalanine (an essential amino acid found in protein) into a form that can be used by the body. Both breast and cow's milk cause phenylalanine and its by-products to accumulate in the child's body, preventing normal brain development.

Lofenalac (Mead Johnson) is a special formula for PKU. Its protein source is hydrolyzed casein; its carbohydrate source is corn syrup and tapioca starch; its fat source is corn oil.

ELECTROLYTE IMBALANCE

A metabolism malfunction whereby protein carbohydrates and fats are not properly broken down can cause an acid condition, which can critically deplete a child's alkali reserves. Formulas for electrolyte imbalance—used also in cases of dehydration associated with diarrhea or vomiting—are prescribed cautiously and usually used as temporary treatment.

Lytren (Mead Johnson) and *Pedialyte* (Ross) are two electrolyte imbalance formulas. They contain no protein, fat, or vitamins A and D. (*Pedialyte* contains no phosphorus.) *Lytren* uses corn syrup solids and glucose for carbohydrates, and *Pedialyte* uses dextrose.

SODIUM RESTRICTION

Some infants, because of fluid retention, require low-sodium formulas. *Lonalac* (Mead Johnson) is such a formula. It also does not contain vitamins D or C.

HIGH-PROTEIN—HIGH-CALORIE REQUIREMENT

Premature infants often need formulas of increased nutrient density because of their inability to consume large enough amounts of ordinary formulas.

Premature Formula (Mead Johnson), *Probana* (Mead Johnson), and *Similac PM 60/40* (Ross) provide high-density protein and calories.

CARBOHYDRATE AND/OR FAT RESTRICTION

In situations where carbohydrates and fats must be restricted, *CHO-Free Formula Base* (Syntex), *Pregestimil* (Mead Johnson), and fortified skim milk are the formulas advised. Syntex's *CHO-Free Formula Base* is the only one of the three with no carbohydrates, and skim milk is the only one of these with no fat.

77. Any questions about chapter VII?

I'm feeding the same formula to my son as I did to my two daughters, but he doesn't seem to go at it with the same gusto. Are there any differences between formulas for girls and boys?

No, but studies have shown that girls are more responsive than boys to formulas that have a sweeter taste (ones that contain sucrose and corn syrup instead of lactose). Also, low-birth-weight infants are less responsive than their heftier counterparts to the sweeter formulas. As long as your son is gaining weight and is healthy, don't worry about it. All kids—even those of the same sex in the same family—have different tastes, personalities, and eating habits.

Is it bad for a baby's digestive system to let him go to sleep with his bottle?

Babies often fall asleep when nursing, and as long as they're burped afterward, there's no digestive problem. But there is a problem in letting your child use the bottle as a pacifier. When a baby naps or falls asleep with a bottle containing sugary liquids, such as formula, juice, or milk, the sugars in the liquid are fermented by the bacteria on the teeth and can cause decay and other dental problems. Continually using a bottle as a pacifier can cause teeth to be pushed out of position.

CHAPTER VIII

The Myths and Magic of Milk

78. Milk facts that moms (and dads) should know

- Sunlight, bright daylight, and fluorescent light reduce vitamins B_2, B_6, and C in milk.
- Milk should be refrigerated at temperatures 45° F. or below soon after purchase.
- Homogenized milk forms softer curds in the stomach, which aids digestion.
- Whole milk can be frozen (for a year) and thawed in the refrigerator, but it often develops an oxidized flavor that kids don't like. (Also, freezing reduces vitamin B_1 and vitamin C levels in dairy products.)
- Vitamin A must be added to low-fat, skim, and nonfat milk, since the original vitamin is removed with the milk fat during processing.
- Vitamin D is added to most fluid milks but not all; so check the labels. (When vitamin D is added, it must be 400 IU per quart.)
- Evaporated milk must be refrigerated once it's opened— and should be transferred to a clean container.
- Acidophilus milk is pasteurized low-fat or skim milk cultured with a friendly bacteria called *Lactobacillus acidophilus,* which helps maintain the microorganism balance in the intestinal tract and helps replace necessary bacteria that are lost after antibiotic treatment.
- Imitation milk and milk products are not recommended for feeding infants and young children.
- Milk that remains open in the refrigerator often takes on other food odors, but it's still safe to drink.
- Antibiotics, such as penicillin, should not be taken with milk.

- Seventy-seven percent of the U.S. dietary consumption of calcium and 66 percent of the Canadian consumption comes from milk.
- There is now a lactase tablet (and liquid) for children with a lactose intolerance that can be added directly to milk, which will allow the child not only to drink milk but to eat foods like yogurt and cottage cheese as well.

79. How much milk do kids really need?

For the first year of life, a child's diet is primarily milk, which provides the necessary nutrients for this rapid period of growth. Around two and during the preschool years, the growth rate slows and energy requirements are less, although calcium and other vitamins and minerals are needed nonetheless for developing bones, tissues, and teeth. Two 8-oz. glasses a day are sufficient during your child's second year, a time when many children turn off milk; but it's advisable to compensate for this by providing other dairy products, such as cheese, milk puddings, and yogurt. (See section 81, Delicious Treats That Even Milk-Haters Love.) Once the "terrible twos" are over, most kids will increase their consumption of milk, but some don't do so until five or six—and others never do.

- A child needs three (8-oz.) servings of milk a day. (A child under eight years of age can use 6-oz. servings.)
- A teenager needs four (8-oz.) servings of milk a day.

Calcium needs are greatest during adolescence (a period when girls have been found to have poorer nutrient intakes than boys); but one quart of milk daily, or its equivalent in other milk products, will provide all the calcium and more than half the protein recommended for teenagers, as well as substantial amounts of vitamins A and B_2, and the recommended allowance of vitamin D.

80. How do substitutes stack up?

I've met parents who think that a child is getting enough calcium in his diet if he eats ice cream twice a day! Needless to say, this isn't so. Two scoops of vanilla ice cream (about a cup) supply only 194 mg. calcium. The RDA for children is between 800 and 1,200 mg. daily, which three to four servings of milk adequately supply—*without* antinutrients like refined sugar (which can destroy nutrients) and with half the calories.

One cup of whole cow's milk has 288 mg. of calcium. With this in mind, here are some substitutes to evaluate for use in your child's meals:

Other Milks	Calcium (per cup)
Goat's milk	315 mg.
Skim milk	296 mg.
Low-fat milk	276 mg.
Buttermilk	296 mg.
Evaporated milk (Unsweetened and not reconstituted)	635 mg.
Evaporated milk (sweetened and not reconstituted)	802 mg.
Dry whole milk	1,164 mg.
Dry no-fat milk	1,570 mg.
Nonfat instant milk	1,177 mg. (3.2-oz. envelope)
Plain whole milk yogurt	272 mg.
Plain skim milk yogurt	294 mg.

Cheeses	Calcium (per oz.)
American (processed)*	174 mg.
Cheddar	204 mg.
Cottage (creamed)	136 mg.
Cream cheese	23 mg.
Fontina	156 mg.
Mozzarella	147 mg.
Mozzarella (low-moisture)	163 mg.
Muenster	203 mg.
Swiss	272 mg.
Swiss (pasteurized process)	219 mg.
Whole-milk Ricotta	514 mg. (per cup)

* Has high sodium content.

Other Foods	*Calcium (per cup)*
Brussels sprouts	50 mg.
Raw Cabbage	74 mg.
Cashew nuts	53 mg.
Green Beans	81 mg.
Lettuce (Romaine)	37 mg.
Canned salmon (with bones)	431 mg.
Hulled sunflower seeds	174 mg.
Egg (medium)	24 mg. (per egg)

81. Delicious treats that even milk-haters love

Adding milk and milk products to different foods in enticing ways is far better for parents and children than getting into arguments over what's left undrunk in the glass. You can't fool milk-haters all of the time, but you can fool them *some* of the time. A little here and a little there adds up to delicious, sufficient milk nutrition.

For breakfast

DANDI SCRAMBLES
(1 serving = approx. 82 mg. calcium)

2 eggs
1 scant tbsp. butter or fortified margarine

¼ cup cottage cheese
salt and pepper to taste

Beat eggs. Melt butter in frying pan and pour in eggs. As they begin to set, add cottage cheese and then scramble in pan until done. Add salt and pepper. (One serving)

For lunch

MUENSTER MONSTER SANDWICH
(1 serving = approx. 213 mg. calcium)

1½ tbsp. peanut butter (natural)
½ tbsp. mayonnaise
2 slices whole wheat bread

3 thin slices of muenster cheese
Lettuce

Thin peanut butter with mayonnaise and spread on bread. Add muenster and lettuce, cut sandwich in quarters. (Don't ask me why, but kids like it better this way.)

For fun

SUNSHINE SHERBERT
(1 serving = approx. 111 mg. calcium)

3½ tbsp. honey
¾ cup canned fruit (unsweetened)
1½ cups buttermilk

1 tbsp. lemon juice
grated lemon rind (from whole fresh lemon)
2 egg whites

Put honey and fruit in blender on low speed. Add buttermilk, lemon juice and rind. Blend thoroughly and then pour into freezer tray. Freeze until firm. Meanwhile, beat egg whites until stiff. When honey-and-fruit mixture is ready, put into bowl, beat well, and fold in egg whites. Return entire mixture to freezer. In an hour or two it will make a super dessert. (Four servings)

HONEY HEAVEN
(1 serving = approx. 296 mg. calcium)

1 cup skim (or low-fat) milk
1 tsp. honey

¾ tsp. vanilla
cinnamon

Warm milk, honey, and vanilla, then pour quickly in blender to froth. Serve and sprinkle with cinnamon. (One serving)

BANANA BEAUTY
(1 serving = approx. 296 mg. calcium)

2 sliced ripe bananas
¼ cup orange juice
dash of vanilla

2 cups reconstituted nonfat dry milk (but substitute 1 cup ice cubes for each cup water)

Put ingredients into blender—adding ice slowly—and blend until sloshy and yummy. (Two to three servings)

82. Yogurt is more than yummy

An excellent source of easily assimilated, high-quality protein, yogurt does a lot more than simply taste good. Many physicians recommend it for children who are taking antibiotics because antibiotics wipe out friendly and unfriendly bacteria indiscriminately—which often causes diarrhea. Yogurt can put the friendly bacteria back into the intestinal tract.

> *Yogurt is particularly good for children
> who have difficulty in digesting milk.*

But not all yogurts that are on the market will do the trick. If you want to test a brand to see if it contains the necessary live cultures, use a couple of tablespoons of it as a starter for making your own.

To test yogurt
> Mix a few tablespoons of the plain yogurt with a cup of warmed (not boiled) milk. Leave the mixture overnight in a warm place (over the pilot light on the range will do). If your yogurt passed the test and had live cultures, the milk will have thickened somewhat by morning. If your yogurt failed, the milk will just be . . . milk. (If so, change your brand.)

Yogurt is particularly good for children who have difficulty in digesting milk. Because the lactose in yogurt is partially broken down by the fermenting process, children with lactose intolerance can often enjoy it as a fine source of calcium.

Like milk, yogurt is a prime supplier of calcium, vitamin B_2 (riboflavin), and protein. (It also contains vitamin A, C, B_1, niacin, and iron.) And cup for cup, it can count toward your child's recommended milk allowance (see section 79).

To keep yogurt tasting tasty, keep it refrigerated at 40° F. or lower. (It can maintain its flavor for ten days or longer this way.) When yogurt remains at higher temperatures—or for a really long time in the refrigerator—it usually develops a sharp flavor that kids don't respond to. It's still edible, however. Just stir the liquid that has separated back into the yogurt or discard it. Fruit-flavored yogurt can be frozen up to six weeks; thawing takes about three hours at room temperature. (Plain yogurt does not freeze well.)

MAKE YOUR OWN YOGURT

Heat one quart of fresh skim milk until it is hot but not boiling.

Stir in one cup of powdered skim milk, plus three tablespoons of ready-made yogurt.

Pour mixture into a wide-mouthed thermos, cover, and let stand overnight. (It takes about six hours for yogurt to achieve the right consistency.)

In the morning, remove the top of the thermos and put the yogurt in the refrigerator.

HOW TO GET YOGURT-HATERS TO LOVE (OR AT LEAST TRY) IT

THE BREAKFAST SPECIAL

Flavor plain yogurt with a dash of vanilla (or any other flavoring your child likes) and serve it over ready-to-eat breakfast cereal.

THE YOGI HOAGIE

(This can be messy, but kids love things that they can make themselves.)

Slice a banana in half lengthwise and spread each half lightly with yogurt—then put together for a finger-licking treat.

THE ORANGE FREEZY

2 cups low-fat yogurt	2 tsps. vanilla
1 small can frozen concentrated orange juice	

Combine ingredients. Mix well and put in ice cube tray— or small individual paper cups—to freeze.

83. Any questions about chapter VIII?

*My child is allergic to milk, which prevents me from making
many desserts, cakes, and sauces that I used to prepare for
the rest of my family. Are there substitutes for milk that can
be used in these recipes?*

Yes, there are. You can purchase milk substitutes made
from soy. Soy "milks" work well in many recipes. They can
be drunk as a beverage, too, but most children do not take to
their taste easily. (See section 115.)

If your child has a lactose intolerance, you should ask your
doctor about a new lactase tablet—also available in liquid
form—that can convert lactose into a highly digestible simple
sugar and allow your child to enjoy a variety of dairy products, including cottage cheese, yogurt, and whole milk.

CHAPTER IX

There's More to Feeding Baby Than Holding the Spoon

84. Starting solid foods

Mothers are usually impatient to start an infant on solid foods, but according to the American Academy of Pediatrics, "justification for this practice appears to rest on opinion, rather than on demonstrated proof of benefit or harm." The academy adds that "no nutritional advantage or disadvantage has yet been proven for supplementing adequate milk diets with solid foods in the first three or four months of life." A mother who starts her child too early on solid foods runs the risk of satisfying the infant with foods of an inferior nutritional content, while decreasing his intake of needed nutritious milk.

> *Starting too early can be risky.*

Don't be in a rush to fill up your baby. The need for additional nutrients in the baby's diet comes around two and a half to three and a half months of age, when the need for iron and vitamin B_1 (thiamine) increases. Trying to force solids on a child who does not need them and is not ready for them, in the hope that it will help him sleep through the night, is foolish, possibly harmful, and doesn't work.

There may be circumstances in which a doctor feels it is necessary to put your child on solids early; but if not, the generally accepted schedule is:

Age	Food
2½–3 months	cereal and/or fruit (some doctors recommend starting with fruit because babies seem to prefer it to cereal)
3½–4½ months	vegetables
4½–5½ months	meat
6 months	egg yolk

85. Solid facts

- Eggs are one of the foods most likely to cause allergy. If there is a history of allergies in the family, it's best to wait until the child is over eight months before starting egg yolk. (The white should not be included when starting, since it's the white that usually causes the allergic reaction.)
- When starting cereals, begin with rice. Wheat causes allergic reactions more often than other cereals.
- The best cereals—the ones with the most protein roughage and vitamins—are whole wheat and oatmeal.
- Avoid corn starch puddings and gelatin desserts. (Corn starch has little nutritive value, and gelatin desserts are overloaded with sugar.)
- Since babies get enough starch in their cereals (usually served twice a day), don't buy commercial fruits and vegetables that also contain starch. (Check the labels!)
- Before giving a child any commercially prepared mixture of meats and vegetables, be sure he's tasted each food separately; otherwise any allergic reaction cannot be pinpointed. (Offer one new food every five or six days.)
- Don't add salt or sugar to baby's food. An infant's taste buds are undeveloped and don't need either.
- Be sure to check the safety button on the jar lid when buying baby food. It should be sunken if the vacuum formed by commercial sterilization is intact, and you should hear a pop when you open the jar. If the safety button is raised before you open the jar, it indicates an imperfect seal, and the food should not be given to your child.
- Leftover juices and fruits can be kept in the refrigerator for three days; strained vegetables, meats, and desserts

will keep fresh for two days—*provided that you've* not *fed these foods from the jars!* (The salivary amylase, an enzyme in saliva, gets into the food and breaks down starch—and any bacteria in the baby's mouth can encourage the growth of other, potentially harmful, bacteria.)

- The top name-brand baby food companies (Gerber, Beech-Nut, and Heinz) have recently removed all preservatives, artificial colors, artificial flavors, nitrates, nitrites, and MSG from their foods. (Check labels nonetheless.) Although most have also removed salt, they still use modified starch in many products.

86. Catering to baby's invisible sweet tooth

> *Sugar is where you least expect it.*

Though commercial baby food manufacturers have drastically reduced the sugar in their products, sugar is still present in desserts and in some foods where parents least expect it.

Heinz's "Mixed Cereal with Apples & Bananas," "Oatmeal with Apples & Bananas," "Rice Cereal with Apples & Bananas" all have 6 percent added sugar.

Beech-Nut's "Cera-Meal" (balanced meals for infants) all contain some lactose and corn syrup.

Gerber's "Toddler Meals"—Beef & Rice with Tomato Sauce, Chicken Stew, Green Beans, Potatoes & Ham Casserole, Spaghetti & Meat Balls, Vegetable & Turkey Casserole—all contain some sugar, as do their "Finger Foods"—Chicken Sticks, Meat Sticks, and Turkey Sticks.

(In most baby foods that include bacon, the bacon has been cured with some sugar.)

87. Baby's food allergies

Allergies can be caused by many substances, and they often tend to run in families (although the substance—or offending allergen—might differ). The food ingredients that are often included in babies' diets and are most likely to prompt allergic reactions are milk, citrus fruit, egg, corn, gluten, and wheat.

Symptoms of Food Allergies: Eczema, skin rashes of various sorts, vomiting, diarrhea, persistent cough, persistent runny nose.

Before diagnosing and treating any allergy, check with a nutritionally oriented doctor. (What might appear to be an allergy to milk could, in fact, be caused by an antibiotic given to the cow from which the milk was taken!)

Heinz, Gerber, and Beech-Nut all offer lists of their baby foods with complete allergenic information. Write to:

> Consumer Relations Department
> Heinz U.S.A.
> P.O. Box 57
> Pittsburgh, Pennsylvania 15230
>
> Gerber Products Company
> Fremont, Michigan 49412
>
> Beech-Nut Products
> P.O. Box 127
> Fort Washington, Pennsylvania 19034

(Beech-Nut also has a nutrition Hot Line to answer any feeding question. The toll-free number is 1-800-523-6633.)

88. Making your own baby food is easier than you thought

It's not that difficult to make your own baby food. All you need is a blender, liquid (fruit juice, milk, water, soup), and you can puree family leftovers (unseasoned) into nutritious gourmet baby meals.

BABY PATÉ

¼ lb. chicken livers
¼ cup unseasoned chicken broth (or water)

Good Source:
Iron, calcium, vitamin A

Put livers and broth in saucepan, bring to boil, and then reduce heat. Simmer for eight minutes. Pour into a blender (liver and liquid) and blend to desired consistency. (For children over six months, you can add a tablespoon of diced onion to the liquid for flavor.)

CREAMY AVOCADO SOUP

¼ large ripe avocado
½ cup milk

Good Source:
Potassium, calcium, vitamins A, B, C, D, E, and K

Put avocado pulp in a blender, turn on low speed, and slowly add milk. (Add more or less milk for consistency desired.) Heat to serving temperature.

CHICKEN SUPREME

¼ cup cooked chicken (no skin)
¼ cup cooked asparagus
¼ cup white sauce (see below)

Good Source:
Calcium, iron, vitamin A, and potassium

Puree chicken and asparagus in blender (use milk if liquid is necessary for proper blending). Put in bowl and mix in *White Sauce:*

1 tbsp. butter (or margarine)   ¾ cup milk
1 tbsp. flour

Melt butter in saucepan and stir in flour (with a wire whisk) before butter browns. Heat milk almost, but not quite, to boiling point. Keep stirring flour and butter, and add the heated milk all at once. Let the mixture come to a boil and thicken. Simmer for two to four minutes. Sauce will keep, if refrigerated, for four days; it can be used with any pureed leftovers.

BABY BERRY DELIGHT

¼ cup strawberries
⅔ tbsp. apple juice
A few drops of honey
¼ cup yogurt

Good Source:
Vitamin C and calcium

Blend first three ingredients, then strain out seeds. (For older children, seeds can remain.) Mix with yogurt.

89. Any questions about chapter IX?

Can I heat my daughter's baby food in a microwave oven? Will it destroy the vitamins in the food?

Actually, heating baby food in a microwave oven destroys fewer vitamins than heating the food by conventional methods. (Microwaves penetrate the food, causing moisture molecules to vibrate, which results in friction that produces heat. Since some microwaves hit the food directly and others bounce off the oven, it's best to stir the food midway during heating.) You can heat the baby food in a glass dish or right in the jar. (Make sure the lid is *not* on the jar when you place it in the microwave.) Use a medium setting. For a 4½-oz. jar of strained food, the time would be fifteen to twenty-five seconds. For a 7½-oz. jar of junior food, the time would be about twenty to thirty seconds. Be sure not to overheat and to stir the contents during cooking and before serving to evenly distribute the heat. *Test the temperature of the food before serving it to your child.*

CHAPTER X

Time for Table Food

90. What are balanced meals?

Basically, a cross between a myth and an endangered species. Balanced meals and diets are written about, talked about—and rarely found on dinner tables. Food processing, soil depletion, chemical additives, and other by-products of technological advance have robbed so many nutrients from food that even diligent parents have a hard time providing their children with a healthy distribution of vitamins and minerals.

Take a simple item like bread, for instance. Practically all brands you find in today's supermarket have been "enriched." Now that *sounds* great, but what "enriched" means is that the twenty-two natural nutrients that should be in the bread but aren't, which were lost in processing, have been replaced by three B vitamins, vitamin D, calcium, and iron salts. You have to admit that's a pretty poor balancing act right there.

> *No matter how nutritious any food is,*
> *it cannot supply all the nutrients.*

Nonetheless, planning your child's meals intelligently *is* important because vitamins, minerals, and a child's metabolism work best when they're all kept nutritionally in tune. Vitamin A works best with B complex, vitamin D, vitamin E, calcium, phosphorus, and zinc. Translated into foods, this means that a child who eats a tuna fish sandwich with lettuce on whole wheat bread, with a glass of milk, is getting optimum vitamin-mineral efficiency.

Children have a tendency to go through monofood periods, where they'll favor one food above all others and tend to eat it to the exclusion of others. No matter how nutritious that food is, it cannot supply *all* the nutrients the child needs.

- Nutrients work together in teams.
- One nutrient cannot make up for a shortage of another.
- Foods from the four basic food groups should be eaten each day.
- Variety in a child's diet is the best defense against overconsumption or deficiency of any nutrient.

91. The four food groups—and what your child needs from each

To plan a balanced diet for your child, you need to become familiar with the four basic food groups and the recommended number of portions that should be eaten from them each day.

MILK GROUP

Primarily supplies calcium, protein, and vitamin B_2 (riboflavin)

All types of milk (used in foods or as beverages); yogurt, ice cream,* ice milk; natural, processed,† cottage, and other cheeses.
3 servings per day for a child
4 servings per day for a teenager

* High sugar content.
† High sodium content.

MEAT GROUP

Primarily supplies protein, iron, niacin, and vitamin B_1 (thiamine)

Beef, veal, pork, lamb, fish, poultry, liver, or eggs. Dried peas, beans, soy extenders, and nuts combined with animal protein—including eggs, milk, and cheese—or grain protein can be substituted for meat serving.
2 servings per day for children and teenagers

FRUIT-VEGETABLE GROUP

Primarily supplies vitamins A and C.

Citrus fruits, tomatoes, cabbage, leafy green and orange vegetables; potatoes, other vegetables, and fruits.
4 servings per day for children and teenagers

GRAIN GROUP

Primarily supplies vitamin B_1 (thiamine), iron, and niacin.

Whole or enriched grains—barley, buckwheat, corn, oats, rice, rye, wheat—and all breads, hot or cold cereals, macaroni, noodles, and other pasta.
4 servings per day for children and teenagers

92. How big is a serving?

Serving sizes are individually determined. A smaller, less active child will eat a smaller serving; teenagers require larger servings.
As a guide

- In the milk group, 1 cup is considered a serving for all whole, skim, or reconstituted milk, as well as for yogurt, buttermilk, and cottage-type cheese. A serving of hard cheese is usually 1 oz.
- In the meat group, a serving is approximately 2 to 3 oz.
- In the fruit and vegetable group, 1 whole fresh fruit, or ½ cup canned fruit is considered a serving; ½ cup is the approximate size of a cooked vegetable serving.
- In the grain group, a slice of bread is considered 1 serving. For pasta and cereal the serving size is ½ cup.

93. Why breakfast is important

Breakfast comes after the longest period during which your child has been without food. It's the prime nutritional charge that kids—especially teenagers—need in order to cope successfully with the physical and emotional energy stresses of the day.

- It raises blood-sugar levels, which can drop during the night.
- It supplies the brain and body with the nutrients necessary for proper learning. (Studies have shown that kids who skip breakfast perform at a lower level in school.)
- It cannot be compensated for by a good lunch or dinner.

94. What's in those cereal boxes?

The best thing I can say about ready-to-eat cereals is that they're usually served with milk. Granted that they're members of the grain food group (although in dubious standing) and that they're convenient to serve at a time of day when family members are rushing to get out of the house, but they are far from being the providers of supernutrition that their manufacturers claim them to be.

Grains—oats, wheat, corn, rice, and others—are naturally high in nutrients. But the heat processing and toasting of most ready-to-eat cereals deplete natural nutrients, and the addition of other ingredients—such as soy flour and sugar—adversely affects the natural goodness even more.

Don't be fooled by "enriched" cereals. Enriching merely means that some (*not all*) of the nutrients lost during processing have been replaced.

> *Just because a cereal is fortified doesn't mean your child will be able to use the vitamins.*

What about "fortified" cereals, you ask? Fortification is the addition of vitamins and minerals not necessarily found in that grain or in amounts larger than would naturally be there. Although reason might tell you that's terrific—which is what the manufacturers want it to tell you—the fact is that just because a vitamin or mineral is added to a food does not mean that the vitamin or mineral will be used by your child's body. A recent study done by Consumers Union shows that "there is no consistent connection between added vitamins and minerals and nutritional quality of breakfast cereals."

Probably the worst thing about these boxed breakfasts is their sugar content. (Only Shredded Wheat and Grape-Nuts have no *added* sugar, which doesn't mean that they're sugar-free.) The next to worst thing is a toss-up between their sodium content and their additives. Most cereals have a sodium content averaging 227 mg. per serving (except for Shredded Wheat, Frosted Mini-Wheats, and most granola cereals, which contain 50 mg. or less). As for additives, BHT and BHA (antioxidants to keep the cereals fresh) are present in more than half the cereals on the market, and artificial colors and flavors are rampant in children's presweetened cereals.

95. Making the best of a bad situation

Even a breakfast of low-nutrition cereal is better for your child than no breakfast at all. And there are a few things you can do to accentuate the positives and reduce the negatives.

- Make sure that your child eats the cereal with milk (Consumers Union's study showed that many kids don't).
- Add fresh fruit to the cereal.
- Mix yogurt and strawberries (or other high-vitamin-C fruit) and serve atop dry cereal as a treat.
- Buy unsweetened cereal and add your own sugar, if absolutely necessary (1 level teaspoon added to an ounce of cereal is way below the amount of sugar in those that have been presweetened).
- Don't add salt to hot cereals when cooking before checking to see if salt has already been added to the cereal mix.
- Add powdered milk to the cooking water for hot cereals.
- Select the lesser of the sugar-evil cereals.

96. Not-so-sweet mysteries about cereals revealed

PERCENTAGE OF SUGAR BY WEIGHT

Cereal	Percent of sugar	Cereal	Percent of sugar
All Bran	19	Honey Comb	37
Alpha Bits	38	Kix	5
Apple Jacks	55	Life	16
Cap'n Crunch	40	Lucky Charms	42

Cereal	Percent of sugar	Cereal	Percent of sugar
Cheerios	3	Oatmeal	0
Chex	4	100% Bran	21
Cocoa Pebbles	43	Product 19	10
Cocoa Puffs	33	Quaker 100%	
Concentrate	9	Natural Cereal	21
Cookie Crisp	44	Raisin Bran	30
Corn Flakes	5	Rice Krispies	8
Count Chocula	40	Shredded Wheat	1
Crazy Cow	40	Special K	5
C.W. Post	29	Sugar Frosted Flakes	41
Farina	0	Sugar Smacks	56
40% Bran	13	Super Sugar Crisp	46
Frankenberry	44	Total	8
Froot Loops	48	Trix	36
Frosted Mini-Wheats	26	Wheatena	0
Fruity Pebbles	43	Wheat Germ	0
Golden Grahams	30	Wheaties	8
Grape-Nuts	7		

97. How to convert nonbreakfast-eaters

> *Don't use breakfast time to discipline
> your child.*

Most kids who skip breakfasts have parents who skip breakfasts or grab a doughnut and coffee and rush off to work. If you want your kids to eat right, it's important to set a good example—and once you start, you'll find you feel a lot better for it yourself.

It's not easy to break a child of a negative habit, but it's not impossible either.

Here are some things you can try:

- Offer foods that you don't ordinarily serve for breakfast. (If your child loves peanut butter sandwiches for lunch, the novelty of having one for breakfast might jump-start his appetite.)

- Cut a slice of cheese into strips and make the child's initial on a piece of whole wheat bread. Place it under the broiler until cheese melts. (Kids respond well to anything with their initials on it.)
- Blender drinks with milk, a fresh fruit or berries, a tablespoon or two of protein powder, and ice cubes look like treats when served with straws. (Perfect for teenagers whose usual excuse for skipping breakfast is that they have no time for a meal.)
- Wake your child earlier so that there isn't appetite-killing stress about being late for school.
- *Don't* use breakfast time to criticize, discipline, or argue with your child. (If someone scolded you every morning when you walked into the kitchen, you wouldn't have much of an appetite either.)
- *Don't* make an issue out of any food. Nature's pantry offers a wide selection of foods with equivalent nutrient values. (See section 100.)
- *Don't* ask your child *if* he wants breakfast; ask if he wants eggs or cereal. (Even better, have a breakfast waiting on the table. Mornings are times when many children are not prepared to make decisions and are relieved when they have already been made.)
- Appeal to the child's sense of humor by serving cereal in a container other than the usual bowl—something outrageously large (a punch bowl) —or divide the portion into three small cups and make up a "tasting-the-three-bears'-porridge" game.
- Explain to your child how the foods he eats now can affect his health as an adult. (Kids are actually more interested in their own well-being than parents give them credit for.)

98. School lunches

In *theory*, school lunches are nutritionally balanced meals; in *fact*, they are so nutritionally poor that they're virtually hazardous to a growing child's health. There are a few exceptions, but only a few, and only because concerned parents have banded together and pressed for the changes.

As a rule, school cafeterias serve meals that are low in

fiber, high in refined carbohydrates and sugars, and surfeited with processed, vitamin-depleted foods. And to add insult to your child's nutritional injury, the meals taste awful, too.

> *Some of the poorest nutritional habits*
> *are learned in school.*

Many schools also sell candy, gum, soft drinks, and artificially flavored ice bars. It's difficult to explain to a child that these foods are bad for him when they're being sold in a place of learning that's supposed to be good for him.

It might be convenient to have your child eat at school, but is it worth handicapping his learning? A high-sugar intake at lunch can cause a drop in blood sugar during the afternoon, which can in turn leave your child fatigued, inattentive, and unable to retain what's being taught. Excessive sugar can also prompt delinquency. (See section 103.)

99. Some of the best lunches come in brown bags

It's not difficult to prepare nutritious lunches for your child, and with the right planning, you can do it ahead of time—and without having to resort to expensive, nonnutritive processed luncheon meats.

TEN LUNCHES THAT KEEP KIDS AND WORKING MOTHERS IN MIND

1. Cottage cheese and pineapple (unsweetened) sandwich on nut bread/carrot sticks/sunflower seeds/milk.
2. Tuna salad with lettuce in pita bread/cherry tomatoes/pear or peach/milk.
3. Peanut butter and sliced apple sandwich/carrot strips/orange slices/milk.
4. Cottage cheese and raisin sandwich on banana bread/green pepper slices/tangerine/milk.
5. Chicken salad with chopped celery in pita bread/apple/milk.
6. Chopped egg (mixed with a little mayonnaise, grated onion, and carrot)/peanuts/grapes/milk.

7. Baked beans (mashed with a little onion and home-made chili sauce) in pita bread/cucumber strips/melon slices or cubes/milk.

8. Yogurt with fruit (can be put in wide-mouthed thermos)/granola/carrot strips/juice.

9. Vegetable soup (in wide-mouthed thermos)/cheese/crackers/peach/milk.

10. Salmon salad with chopped celery on whole wheat bread/sunflower seeds or peanuts/banana/milk.

Sandwiches can be kept frozen (wrapped in foil) and taken out when the child is ready to go to school. (Lettuce and other greens should not be frozen. They can be added when the sandwich is taken out of the freezer.)

Use low-fat milk in place of whole milk. (There's usually enough fat in a child's diet.)

100. Why your child doesn't have to eat spinach or liver

Just because Popeye eats spinach doesn't mean that your child has to. There are enough nutrients in alternative foods to compensate for the one your child doesn't like.

If Your Child Doesn't Like . . .	Prime Source of . . .	Alternatives Listed in Section . . .
Liver	Vitamin A	8
	Vitamin B_1	9
	Vitamin B_2	10
	Vitamin B_6	11
	Vitamin B_{12}	12
	Biotin	16
	Pantothenic Acid	18
	Choline	19
	Folic Acid	23
	Inositol	24
	Niacin	26
	Copper	36
	Iron	39

If Your Child Doesn't Like . . .	Prime Source of . . .	Alternatives Listed in Section . . .
Spinach	Vitamin A	8
	Vitamin B_2	10
	Vitamin E	21
	Folic Acid	23
	Calcium	32
	Iron	39
	Potassium	44
Fish	Vitamin B_2	10
	Vitamin D	20
	Niacin	26
	Calcium	32
	Copper	36
	Phosphorus	43
	Selenium	45
Eggs	Vitamin A	8
	Vitamin B_2	10
	Vitamin B_6	11
	Vitamin B_{12}	12
	Biotin	16
	Choline	19
	Vitamin E	21
	Folic Acid	23
	Vitamin K	25
	Niacin	26
	Iron	39
	Phosphorus	43
	Zinc	49
Meat	Vitamin B_1	9
	Vitamin B_6	11
	Vitamin B_{12}	12
	Pantothenic Acid	18
	Niacin	26
	Iron	39
	Phosphorus	43
	Zinc	49

If Your Child Doesn't Like . . .	Prime Source of . . .	Alternatives Listed in Section . . .
Citrus Fruits	Vitamin C	17
	Magnesium	40
	Potassium	44
Leafy Green Vegetables	Vitamin A	8
	Vitamin B_2	10
	Vitamin C	17
	Choline	19
	Vitamin E	21
	Folic Acid	23
	Vitamin K	25
	Calcium	32
	Magnesium	40
	Potassium	44
Milk	Vitamin A	8
	Vitamin B_1	9
	Vitamin B_2	10
	Vitamin B_6	11
	Vitamin B_{12}	12
	Vitamin D	20
	Calcium	32
	Zinc	49

(more substitutes
in section 80)

101. Any questions about chapter X?

Would you consider pizza and a salad a nutritious meal?

Sure, if the pizza's made with whole-grain flour and no
artificial ingredients. With the cheese on top, you have something from each of the four basic food groups right there and
a good combination of complete and incomplete proteins,
too.

*My child is a poor eater, but whenever he skips a meal, I give
him a vitamin pill. Should I be giving him more than one?*

Vitamins cannot replace food! They can't work properly without food. Just because you give a child vitamins doesn't mean the child is able to use them. And always bear in mind that because a little of one nutrient helps a child doesn't mean that a lot of that nutrient will do more—in fact, it can do just the reverse.

See section 122 on the finicky eater. If your child's appetite doesn't improve in a week, I'd strongly advise you to consult a nutritionally oriented physician.

Part Three

THE
JUNK FOOD
TRAP

CHAPTER XI

There Are No Bad Children, Only Bad Diets

102. What your kids are eating at those fast-food places

A lot of sugar, starch, fat, salt, additives—and calories! Sure, they get protein, vitamins, and minerals, too, but ounce for ounce, munch for munch, and sip for sip, the bad far outweighs the good. Calories should be proportionate to nutrients. When the balance changes, when there are too many calories and two few nutrients, the result is junk food.

> *The most nutritious part of a McDonald's hamburger is the bun!*

BURGERS Fast-food burgers can supply 44 percent of a teenage boy's requirement for protein (67 percent of a seven-to-ten-year-old's). But when you consider that a Big Mac is also supplying 591 calories, 33 grams of fat, 6 *grams* of sugar, and 963 mg. of sodium; that a Burger King Whopper is supplying 660 calories, 41 grams of fat, 9 grams of sugar, and *1,083 mg. of sodium,* that's an awfully high nutritional price to pay for protein. (See section 52.)

SHAKES Well, the good news is they all contain milk or a milk product; the bad news is that they all contain from *8 to 14 teaspoons of sugar* and from *276 to 685 mg. of salt!* A 9-ounce McDonald's shake has 343 calories; a 9-ounce glass of whole milk has only about 178 calories and much more calcium. (You can blend one for your child at home for less than half the price, calories, sugar, and salt—and double the nutritional value.)

FRIES   With fast-food fried potatoes, less is more—in everything but nutrients. At McDonald's, 5½ ounces of fries give your child 542 calories and 117 mg. of sodium. If you make them at home, 9 ounces are only 434 calories with 8 mg. sodium. Potatoes are a fine source of vitamin C, niacin, potassium, phosphorus, and calcium, but your child is being shortchanged on all of them by taking them with those extra grains of salt.

HOT DOGS   No matter where your child eats them, they're not so hot. They're a high-fat, low-protein meat (a cooked hot dog is 55 percent water, 28 percent fat, and less than 17 percent protein). What's worse, hot dogs contain sodium or potassium nitrite. Nitrites combine with substances called amines, which are commonly found in foods, and form nitrosamines, which have been found to be carcinogenic. There is no such thing as a nitrite-free hot dog, since those look-alikes that are nitrite-free must be labeled "uncured cooked sausage." To compound its drawbacks, a hot dog also contains salt, corn syrup, and dextrose. Next time you take your child out to the ball game, bring along a sandwich from home.

PIZZA   Homemade pizza made with whole-wheat flour can be a nutritious blending of complete and incomplete proteins. At a fast-food restaurant, one-half of a 10-inch pizza (about 7¾ oz.) contains 1,281 mg. of sodium, about 6 grams of sugar, and 506 calories. No matter how you slice it, it doesn't add up to great nutrition.

103. The junk food connection

The evidence is in and the findings are virtually irrefutable that there is a definite connection between delinquency and junk food. In a study done by Dr. Derrick Lonsdale at the

Cleveland Medical Center, it was found that adolescents who ate a diet high in junk foods developed symptoms of "marginal malnutrition" similar to the disease beriberi, a severe vitamin B₁ (thiamine) deficiency.

According to Dr. Lonsdale, junk food junkies with thiamine deficiencies often undergo personality changes, sometimes becoming irritable and aggressive. (They also suffer from abdominal pains, restlessness, insomnia, and nightmares.)

> *Children on junk food diets can undergo
> personality changes.*

Dr. Lendon Smith, in his book *Feed Your Kids Right,* also pinpoints carbohydrates as a cause of deviant behavior among children, emphasizing that the increased incidence of hyperactivity and suspected psychological problems of kids can be related to the increased use of sugar.

To compound the problem, most so-called fast foods and commercial sugary snacks contain artificial colors or flavors. Many children have an allergic reaction to these, which is not manifested by a rash or stomach upset or any of the other usual allergic reactions but by a sudden outburst of delinquent behavior caused by a chemical reaction in the brain.

Glucose metabolism varies in children. In some, the eating of sugary foods will produce a normal rise in blood sugar levels, but an hour or two later there will be a severe drop, *below* the original low blood sugar level. It's this plunge that affects the mood-controlling hormones in the brain and results in hyperactive and violent behavior.

104. How sweet it isn't

The average American child is presently consuming about two pounds of sugar a week—and there's nothing sweet I can say about that! Dr. Allan Cott, author of *Problem Foods,* has found that in the treatment of one thousand children suffering from behavior disorders or learning disabilities, a significant percentage were dramatically improved by removing sugar and junk foods from their diets.

> **Your child might be consuming two pounds
> of sugar a week!**

Antinutrients, such as sugar, need B vitamins for metabolization, and a child who consumes large amounts of junk
foods can become drained of his own necessary supply of
these vitamins if they're not replaced daily. But cutting back
a child's sugar intake isn't easy. Today there are at least one
hundred sweet substances identified as sugars in products on
the market, and manufacturers rely on the fact that the average consumer cannot identify them. But you *can* learn how
(and so can your child). What you must become is a sugar
detective.

Here are the basic clues:

- Ingredients on labels ending in "ose" indicate the presence of sugar.
- Honey, corn syrup, corn syrup solids, maple syrup, molasses, and cane syrup, among others, are also sugars.

If you can spot all of these, you'll be taking a giant step in
the right direction.

105. A matter of Hide-and-Sweet

There are certain products in which you expect to find
sugar, such as ice cream and candy bars, but there are others,
like salt, toothpaste, and *vitamins*, that you'd never suspect.
And the percentages can amaze you!

Heinz Tomato Ketchup is 29 percent sugar—which is more
than the 21.4 percent in *Sealtest Chocolate Ice Cream!*

Dannon Blueberry Lowfat Yogurt is 13.7 percent sugars—
which is more than the 8.7 percent in a can of *Coca-Cola!*

If you prepare your child's chicken dinner with *Shake 'N
Bake Barbecue Style,* you've sabotaged an ordinary meal with
a coating that's 51 percent sugar! That's as much as in a
Hershey bar!

Check labels carefully. Commercial peanut butter has sugar
in a greater percentage than you'd imagine. (*Skippy* has 1.2
percent *more* sugar than *Coca-Cola*.) Even medicines are not

immune. I know they say, "It takes a little sugar to make the medicine go down," but there's a lot more than a little in most children's medications.

Some of the worst offenders are chewable vitamins (see section 70), which contain not only sugar but also artificial colorings and flavoring. These additives have been found to promote allergies that result in disruptive and delinquent behavior. (See section 103.)

A TABLE OF SUGAR CONTENTS

Food	Serving Size	Approximate Teaspoons of Sugar per Serving
DRINKS		
Bird's Eye Awake	4 oz.	3
Cola beverages	6 oz.	3½
Ginger ale	6 oz.	5
Hi-C Orange Drink	6 oz.	5
Kool-Aid	8 oz.	6
Orangeade	8 oz.	5
Root beer	10 oz.	4½
Seven-Up	6 oz.	3¾
Tang	4 oz.	4
CANDIES		
Chocolate bar	1½ oz.	2½
Chewing gum	1 stick	½
Chocolate mints	1	2
Gumdrop	1	2
Hard candy	4 oz.	10
Lifesavers	1	⅓
Peanut brittle	1 oz.	3½
CAKES, COOKIES, AND PIES		
Angel food	1 (4-oz. piece)	7
Cheesecake	1 (4-oz. piece)	2
Cherry pie	1 slice	10
Chocolate cake (plain)	1 (4-oz. piece)	6
Chocolate cake (iced)	1 (4-oz. piece)	10
Brownie	1 (¾ oz.)	3

Food	Serving Size	Approximate Teaspoons of Sugar per Serving
CAKES, COOKIES, AND PIES		
Cupcake (iced)	1	6
Chocolate cookie	1	1½
Fig Newtons	1	5
Gingersnaps	1	3
Macaroons	1	6
Oatmeal cookies	1	2
Sugar cookies	1	1½
Chocolate éclair	1	7
Doughnut (plain)	1	3
Doughnut (glazed)	1	6
DAIRY DESSERTS AND OTHERS		
Chocolate pudding	½ cup	4
Ice cream cone	1	3½
Ice cream soda	1	5
Ice cream sundae	1	7
Malted milk shake	1 (10-oz. glass)	5
Tapioca pudding	½ cup	3
Sherbet	½ cup	9

106. Watch out! Caffeine is not just in coffee

I've heard mothers tell their children, "You're not old enough for coffee; it has caffeine," and then hand them a can of *Coca-Cola*. The truth is that there's almost as much caffeine in a 12-oz. can of cola (64.7 mg.) as there is in a cup of instant coffee (66.0 mg.). Soft drinks, such as *Mountain Dew, Mellow Yellow,* and others, also contain caffeine. Check the labels next time you're in the supermarket, you'll be surprised.

Tea is another beverage often given to children, which shouldn't be. There are 46.0 mg. of caffeine in a five-minute brew. And cocoa, which mothers will give to their kids at bedtime, thinking that it will help them to sleep, has 13.0 mg. of the stimulant.

> *Caffeine is a drug and should be
> treated as such.*

Caffeine is a drug, and children become addicted to it the same way adults do. When suddenly deprived of caffeine, a child used to consuming large amounts in chocolate and sodas will evidence symptoms of withdrawal, which include headaches, stomach cramps, irritability, and depression.

Along with putting heavy stress on your child's endocrine system, caffeine

- depletes vitamin B_1 (thiamine) and inositol
- has a diuretic effect that can wash out your child's potassium and zinc and prevent proper assimilation of *calcium* and *iron!*

If your teenager wants a cup of coffee, offer *non*caffeinated "coffees," such as *Pero, Caffix, Roastaroma,* and *Postum.* And if your child wants a cup of tea, there is a wide selection of herb teas available in a variety of pleasing flavors.

It's easier to stop bad habits before they start.

107. How to help your child break the junk-food habit

- Offer juices or milk shakes instead of soda pop.
- Don't keep junk foods in the house.
- Use carob instead of chocolate.
- Offer nuts and raisins instead of candies.
- Keep nutritious snacks (see section 108) available at all times . . . and where the child can reach them.
- Increase the amount of vitamin-C and B-complex foods in his diet (see sections 9 through 17). For older children, a supplement of stress vitamin B complex, 50–100 mg. daily, is advised.
- Pack lunches for trips so that you can avoid stopping at fast-food restaurants.
- Instead of three meals a day, offer four, five, even six smaller ones, to avoid low-blood-sugar levels, which prompt the child's craving for sweets.

- Stock up on *raw* sunflower seeds (do not give to children under four), and encourage your child to eat them when he feels an urge for sweets. Sunflower seeds release glucose from the liver, which rushes to the brain like adrenaline and produces a similar "lift" effect.

> *Get your kids into* sour *instead of* sweet!

- Try cultivating your child's taste for *sour* foods, such as pickles, unsweetened grapefruit, and unsweetened lemonade. A child's taste buds *can* be converted!

108. Snacking can be healthy

Popcorn is a great snack for children, because it's an excellent way to add bulk and fiber to their diet. Instead of salt, sprinkle some debittered yeast (not brewer's yeast) on top. It tastes terrific, and it adds vitamins galore. (Grated cheddar cheese works well, too.)

Fresh fruits are treasure chests of natural vitamins and minerals. Apples supply magnesium, bananas potassium, and all citrus fruits (as well as cantaloupe) are high in vitamin C. They can be dressed up to look like real treats, when sliced and spread with peanut butter; cottage, cream, or ricotta cheese; even yogurt. And don't count out watermelon; it has more iron than any other fruit!

Dried fruits are candy-sweet and good sources of vitamin A (ten dried apricot halves supply more than 3,000 IU) and calcium (raisins have 18 mg. per ounce).

Raw vegetables are not usually a kid's idea of a snack, but when they're spread with peanut butter or cream cheese and presented on a toothpick, they take on a party appeal. (Don't assume that your child won't go for them just because he doesn't respond well to cooked vegetables. Lots of children prefer the crunchy, snacklike taste of raw carrots and green beans.) There's a wide selection of colors, tastes, and vitamins in celery, cauliflower, green pepper, cucumber sticks, turnip strips, and zucchini rounds.

Seeds and nuts—alone or mixed with one another and raisins—are high in nutrients. Pumpkin seeds are a great source of zinc; and except for cashews and Brazil nuts, most are excellent suppliers of unsaturated fatty acids.

Juices, both fruit and vegetable, are low in sugar, high in vitamins, and take on kid-appeal when served with an orange or pineapple slice wedged on the glass. (Colorful straws add attraction to any beverage a child drinks.)

Milk, especially low-fat milk, makes a great shake when mixed in the blender with the child's favorite fruit, some orange juice, and ice. (Fruit plus ¾ cup powdered milk, ½ cup orange juice, and 1½ cups water with a few ice cubes makes a shake that can be drunk on the spot or frozen and eaten as a popsicle.) And homemade eggnog is a high-protein snap: Blend 1 cup of milk, a raw egg, a teaspoon honey, about ¼ teaspoon of vanilla, and a sprinkling of nutmeg.

Cheese and crackers are calcium-rich and a good combination of dairy and grains. Use *whole-grain* crackers. A Ry-Krisp spread with a dollop of peanut butter and a slice of banana is surprisingly filling and fun.

FOR SPECIAL OCCASIONS

- Think about a Birthday Watermelon instead of a Birthday Cake. Take half a watermelon (slice a piece from the bottom so that it can stand without wobbling), decorate with grapes, then put in the candles.
- Hawaiian Kabobs made by putting pieces of fruit on long kabob spears (or you can make smaller ones on tooth-picks). Pineapple-grape-apple-raisin-orange is a nice combination.

> *Herb teas, especially peppermint, make great iced drinks for kids.*

- Apple whip is fun at parties and can be scooped into small paper cups and served like ices. It's simple, too. Just beat 1 cup of thick (unsweetened and better if home-made) apple sauce, 2 egg whites, and 1 tablespoon of honey until it's thick and peaks like whipped cream.
- Nutty banana balls are a natural confection that will add nutrients to any special occasion. They can be stored in

the refrigerator, so make enough. Mix 2 cups peanut butter (natural) with ½ cup carob powder, ½ cup mashed banana, and 4 teaspoons of vanilla. Shape into balls and roll in wheat germ. Keep in refrigerator at least one hour before serving.

- To add natural color to whipped cream without adding chemicals, you can squeeze raw grated vegetables through a square of nylon net (one cut from a pair of hose will work). For pink, grate raw beet. For yellow, grate raw carrot. For green, grate raw spinach. These *pure* vegetable colorings can be stored in the refrigerator in small tightly closed bottles.

109. Any questions about chapter XI?

Instead of snacking on chocolate and potato chips, my daughters chew sugarless gum. Is this a good substitute?

Sugarless gum is as bad as other junk food, as far as I'm concerned. It contains sorbitol and mannitol, which are reputed to be harmless unless eaten in great quantity but often cause diarrhea in even moderate amounts. Besides that, the gum still contains artificial colors and flavoring. Also, chewing for extended periods of time strains the jaw and stimulates the saliva that gets the digestive tract prepared for food it doesn't receive, creating hunger and gastrointestinal problems.

If chewing is what your daughters want, try offering them some raw carrots and celery. They'll be much better, slimmer, and healthier for it.

What's the advantage of carob over chocolate?

Carob, the powdered seed of the carob tree, has a flavor similar to chocolate but contains no theobromine or caffeine—and is much lower in fat.

How can you say that the bun is the most nutritious part of a McDonald's hamburger? What about all the protein in the meat?

And what about all that saturated fat? And sodium (963 mg!)? Sure, the protein is there, but weighed against the cholesterol and sodium content it loses enough nutritional value to make the enriched bun the winner by default.

Part Four

SPECIAL FOODS FOR SPECIAL KIDS

CHAPTER XII

The Allergic Child

110. What an allergy is

An allergy is a hypersensitivity to a specific substance that, in a smaller quantity, does not bother other people. The allergy-causing substance is known as an antigen or an allergen. These antigens and allergens are divided into categories, according to how a child comes in contact with them.

THE FOUR MAIN CATEGORIES

Ingestants—foods and medicines the child swallows.
Inhalants—things the child breathes in from the air (pollen, dusts, cat and dog dander, feathers, etc.).
Contactants—substances that touch the child's body (dyes; materials such as wool, nylon, and others; poison ivy, etc.).
Injectants—substances that are injected into the child (from antibiotics to insect stings).
(Allergic symptoms can also be triggered by emotional stress, changes in weather, and infections.)

111. Types of food allergies

> *Your child may be allergic to his
> favorite food.*

There are two types of food allergies: obvious and hidden.
Obvious food allergies are those that cause your child to break out in a rash, swell, sneeze, wheeze, or feel headachy relatively soon after eating a specific (and many times a not ordinarily eaten) food, such as strawberries, shellfish, or cashew nuts. But eggs, chocolate, and citrus fruits, along

with other common foods, can cause obvious allergic reactions, too.

Hidden food allergies are those whereby the symptoms appear so gradually that the relationship between the food and the reaction is difficult to recognize. (Symptoms may take twelve to forty-eight hours to develop, or they might not develop unless the child eats a lot of the food for several consecutive days.) These types of allergies are usually caused by foods your child eats daily—citrus fruits, chocolate, milk, corn, wheat, sugar, and so on. Surprisingly, hidden food allergies are often caused by your child's favorite food!

112. Possible symptoms of hidden food allergies

Bed-wetting (see section 124)
Persistent colds
Hyperactivity (see section 133)
Recurring nosebleeds
Mouth-breathing
Poor performance in school
Recurrent ear problems
Headaches
Chronic winter cough
Irritability
Dark circles under eyes

Leg and muscle aches
Puffiness in face
Constipation or diarrhea
Fatigue
Wheezing
Spots on the tongue
Twitchiness
Excessive sleeping
Stomachaches
Stuffy nose
Excessive sweating
Poor attention span
Paleness of skin

113. Preventing allergies

There's no sure way to prevent a child from developing an allergy, but certain measures do help.

- Pregnant women who eat a varied, well balanced diet and avoid consuming large quantities of any food that disagrees with them (especially eggs and milk) are less likely to have allergic children. Also, studies have shown that breast-fed babies are less likely to develop allergies.

> *A varied diet is the best protection
> against allergies.*

- When starting your child on solid foods, wait three to five days between the introduction of each new food.
- Avoid giving a child chocolate or cola.
- Don't introduce egg white to your child's diet until he is at least nine months old.
- Once your child has been given a variety of foods, rotate his menus as much as possible. An allergy to a food is more likely to develop if that particular food is eaten every day.

114. Tests for allergies

Skin tests are often inaccurate in detecting food allergies. If you suspect a food of causing your child to have an allergic reaction, eliminate that food from his diet for one to three weeks. If your child's symptoms disappear, you've probably nailed the right culprit. You might want to feed the food to the child again to see if the symptoms reappear, just to make certain.

I advise consulting your child's doctor or a nutritionally oriented pediatrician (see section 171) before embarking on any radical diet changes.

HOW TO GO ABOUT IT AND WHAT TO EXPECT

- Keep a record of your child's symptoms for a few days before eliminating the food from his diet (see sections 115 through 118 for specific foods), and continue the record while the child is on the new regimen.
- Keep up the regimen for seven to twenty-one days.
- Your child might feel worse before he feels better. Withdrawal-type symptoms (headaches, irritability, tiredness) are not uncommon for the first two or three days, but he should feel better by the end of the first week.
- Significant improvement might take the full three weeks.

A full-scale elimination diet—which entails keeping your child away from milk; all dairy products; corn, luncheon meats, citrus fruits; all breads, starches, and cereals (especially those with wheat and corn); foods with added sugar; carbonated beverages; corn and cottonseed oil; and any commercial foods with artificial coloring or additives for three weeks, and then adding a new food back each day to check for reactions—*should not be undertaken without the supervision of a physician.*

115. Milk-free diets

If you're eliminating milk from an allergic child's diet, these are the foods to be excluded:

- All forms of milk (dry, low-fat, evaporated, goat's, yogurt, buttermilk, skim, powdered), even used in small amounts in soups, sauces, gravies, or puddings—unless your child's physician permits trace amounts.
- All cheeses, ice creams, and sherbets (sherbet contains milk solids).
- Pancake and waffles made with milk (commercially prepared mixes usually contain some form of dried milk).
- All commercially baked breads, cakes, doughnuts, and cookies (milk-free breads are available, or you can bake your own).
- Nondairy substitutes, such as *Coffeemate, Cereal Blend, Preem, Cool Whip,* and others that contain caseinate, a milk protein. (*Coffee Rich* and *Mocha Mix* have no casein and can be used on cereal or as a milk substitute in making pancakes and breads. Soy "milks" can also be used.
- All butter and margarines containing milk (you can use corn oil or soy margarines).

(Since milk-allergic children often have reactions to beef, this, too, might have to be excluded. Check with your child's physician.)

116. Egg-free diets

Many commercial mixed foods contain egg; read labels very carefully or avoid commercial mixes altogether.

A child on an egg-free diet should not have noodles, macaroni, marshmallows, meat loaves (made with egg), custards, ice creams, icings, waffles, cakes, or any baked goods with eggs, unless advised otherwise by a physician.

117. Wheat-free diets

Most breads, crackers, cereals, and cookies should be avoided, as well as luncheon meats, hot dogs, chocolate candies, gravies, and sauces.

Since wheat is present in more foods than you suspect, label reading is essential.

Rice crackers and bread made from cornmeal are acceptable.

118. Corn-free diets

This is one of the most difficult foods to eliminate from a child's diet because it's included in different forms in so many foods (as cornstarch, corn oil, corn syrup, and so on). To be safe, avoid mixed foods and also candies, carbonated beverages, chewing gum, peanut butter, pork and beans, puddings, and sherbets.

119. Some things you should know about food allergies

- If you're eliminating chocolate from your child's diet, you should also eliminate cola (most cola drinks come from cola nuts, which are related to cocoa beans).
- Most children with food allergies can, after a period of avoidance, take smaller amounts of the food without having any reaction.
- Food allergies are usually worse in wintertime.
- A child can occasionally eat a food that he's allergic to and evidence no symptoms, but if the food is eaten too often, his tolerance will break down.
- Colicky babies on formula who develop skin rashes and experience persistent runny noses and digestive upsets in their first six months are likely to evidence food-allergy symptoms when consuming large quantities of milk in later childhood.
- A suspected allergy might not come from the food itself but from the plastic container or can that the food comes in.

120. The allergy-prone child

If your child has hypersensitivities *other* than food (to air pollutants, fabrics, or insect bites, for instance), the following suggested food and supplement regimen can help:

Increase these foods
Fish liver oil, citrus fruits and juices, nutritional yeast, liver, soy products, and alfalfa sprouts.

Vitamins and minerals

Vitamin A	5,000–10,000 IU daily, 5 days a week
Vitamin C	100–1,000 mg. daily
Vitamin B complex	25–100 mg. daily
Pantothenic acid	100–300 mg. daily
Vitamin E	50–400 IU daily

121. Any questions about chapter XII?

How accurate are skin tests for food allergies?

Not very. For example, a skin test might show that your child is allergic to eggs, yet he may be able to eat them without experiencing any allergic reaction. I've known parents who have been told that their child's skin test for milk was negative, and later, through a supervised elimination diet, they discovered that milk was the major cause of their son's perennially stuffed nose.

If you suspect that your child has a food allergy, discuss it with a nutritionally oriented doctor (see section 171). There are now new tongue-taste tests that appear to be more accurate and less stressful for children.

I've been told that my child has a lactose intolerance. Is this the same as a milk allergy?

No. A lactose intolerance is a digestive intolerance to the sugar *lactose* in milk. A milk allergy is a hypersensitivity to the protein in milk.

CHAPTER XIII

Kids to Handle with Care

122. The finicky eater

If your child is one of those kids who thinks anything green is yukky, who spends more time pushing a pea around on his plate than you do for the family laundry, and who looks forward to meals with the same enthusiasm as he does to homework, then you have a finicky eater.

The B-complex vitamins can help stimulate a flagging appetite; try to enrich his diet with these by using a little camouflaged nutrition (see section 55). If he likes chicken, bread it with wheat germ. Sprinkle breakfast cereals with iron-rich raisins and dried peaches. Make a salad dressing of peanut butter and mayonnaise, and he might forget about the fact that lettuce is green. Eggs can be added to milk shakes. (See section 108 for eggnog and vitamin-C-rich fruit shakes.)

Suggested vitamins and minerals:
 Vitamin B complex   50–100 mg. daily
 Vitamin C   100–1,000 mg. daily
 Children's multiple-vitamin-mineral supplement with iron
 (5 days a week)

123. The overweight child

Children who are overweight are usually heavy consumers of refined sugars and other carbohydrates, but it has been found that obesity tends to cluster in families. (With one obese parent, a child has a risk of about 40 percent of becoming an obese adult; with two obese parents, the risk jumps to 70 percent.) Still, how much is a result of genetics and how much is a result of family meal-planning and habits is undetermined. I'm inclined to believe that the latter is at fault.

> *Don't insist that your child eat that*
> *last spoonful!*

Don't encourage a bottle-fed baby to finish the last drop of his formula. If he's stopped nursing, he's satisfied. The same holds true for insisting that a child finish the last spoonful in his dish. This type of pressure, day after day, merely contributes to a pattern of overeating. What you should encourage is vigorous exercise on a regular basis. Set aside time (at least one hour after eating) and join your child in a physical activity.

Since overweight children are usually snackers, you might find that several smaller meals (free of sugars and starches) will be easier for the child to live with and lose weight with. This will also help to keep his blood-sugar levels up and prevent an overproduction of insulin, which creates the craving for carbohydrates in the first place.

Calories do count, and you should count those that your child is consuming. You might not realize how much he's eating. (See section 59 for your child's proper caloric needs. One pound is 3,500 calories.)

Never call your child fat. Say something like, "You have a terrific body, why hide it?" (Psychologists have found that kids who are called "fat" believe it's an unalterable fact and therefore fail more often in their attempts at dieting.) In your efforts to help your child lose weight, emphasize *reclaiming* the trim physique or fabulous figure that he or she has naturally.

Overweight children are not *good* eaters; they're just eaters. It's up to you to supply the right foods in the right amounts. (See section 92.) Don't make the child feel as if he's being deprived when you begin changing his diet; the key is to make him feel as if he's getting something better (which he is).

Avoid luncheon meats. (See section 99 for sandwich suggestions.) Make foods more appealing, and once again emphasize those that are rich in the vitamin B complex. Vary his diet—it's usually the food he craves most often that's giving him his "up," his subsequent "down," and the weight problem. (See sections 107 and 108.)

Increase these foods
Wheat germ, raw green and leafy vegetables, liver (if possible), and water. (As a treat, popcorn is a good source of roughage and low in calories. Sprinkle with debittered yeast instead of salt.)

Suggested vitamins
Vitamin B complex 10–50 mg. 1 to 2 times daily

124. The bed-wetter

For years, late bed-wetting (enuresis) was considered an undeniable indication of a child with emotional problems. Confused parents and children were shunted back and forth between analysts searching for reasons, and in most cases the problem remained unsolved. There are still many theories about bed-wetting, but recent studies have shown that diet is a *major* cause of the problem.

> *That glass of milk at bedtime could be the problem.*

In a study done by Dr. James C. Breneman, chairman of the food allergy committee of the American College of Allergists, unsuspected allergies to cow's milk, chocolate, eggs, grain, and citrus fruit can cause bed-wetting by making the child's bladder swell and keeping the outlet from closing properly. Because the allergies also promote a fall in blood sugar, the child sleeps more deeply, and the alert messages from the bladder fail to reach the brain.

Stress cannot be ruled out as a factor, since it, too, can lower a child's blood-sugar level in the same way that an insulin increase caused by a chocolate bar can.

Foods to avoid
All processed foods, sugary or high-carbohydrate foods, milk and all milk products (see section 115 for listings),

chocolate, and any of the other suspect foods mentioned above (until tested), especially at bedtime.

Suggested vitamins and minerals
Calcium (500 mg.) and magnesium (250 mg.) taken with some nonallergy-causing food in early evening.

125. The delinquent

I hold bad diets heavily responsible for bad children. An adolescent whose diet is high in refined sugars, carbohydrates, and processed food not only has a problem but *is* a problem. Soaring and plunging blood-sugar levels have been shown to promote aggressive, antisocial, and often violent behavior. (See section 103.)

It is a recognized fact that at least 75 percent of all criminals have abnormal glucose-tolerance levels.

If your child's behavior has become or is becoming a cause for concern, eliminate all junk foods from his diet as soon as possible. (See section 107.)

Increase these foods
Meat (not fatty), fish, liver, chicken, eggs, milk, leafy green vegetables, whole wheat, peanuts (unsalted), yeast. All foods rich in thiamine (B_1).

Suggested vitamins and minerals
Antistress B complex   50–100 mg. daily
Vitamin C   100–1,000 mg. daily
Children's multiple-vitamin-mineral complex with zinc (1 daily 5–6 days a week).

126. The underachiever

If you know that your child is bright but his marks in school don't show it, the cause might well be his diet. Once again, high sugar and carbohydrate consumption seem to be the culprits.

A recent study of American schoolchildren for a period of five months showed that those who were prohibited from eating refined sugars and grains; restricted to natural additive-free foods; and put on a regimen of supplementary B vitamins, niacinamide, and vitamins A and D increased their IQs by an average of 4.8 points. Compared with a group that was fed candy, the vitamin-supplemented children increased their reading skills to 175 percent above those of the sugar eaters. (It was also noted that absence, tardiness, and disruptive behavior occurred as much as twice as often among the sugar-fed children.)

The first thing to look into if your child is not working up to his potential is his lunchbox. You might also have a hair analysis done to check for toxic mineral levels. (See section 65.)

Increase these foods
Whole grains, brewer's yeast, eggs, milk, meat, fish, poultry, almonds, peanuts, sunflower seeds, green and yellow vegetables (raw or steamed), citrus fruits.

Suggested vitamins and minerals
A children's multivitamin and mineral supplement, which includes zinc (1 daily, 5 days a week)
Calcium   500 mg. daily
Magnesium   250 mg. daily
Vitamin B complex   50–100 mg. daily

127. The clumsy child

There are many reasons for children who are naturally clumsy—atonic musculature, excess weight, emotional problems—but the cause might also be a deficiency of folate in the child's diet.

A study done in Canada by Dr. M. I. Botez of Montreal showed that supplementation of 5 mg. weekly markedly decreased the children's poor coordination.

Folic acid won't turn a *klutz* into a choreographer's delight, but adding more of it to your child's diet might prevent him from being the team's liability.

Increase these foods
Dark green leafy vegetables, egg yolk, carrots, apricots, cantaloupe, whole wheat and dark rye flour.

Suggested vitamins and minerals
Folic acid   200–400 mcg. daily
Vitamin B complex   50–100 mg. daily

128. The liar

All kids fib once in a while, but a child who repeatedly lies is something else. And that something else is not necessarily a bad child, or even a psychologically disturbed one. Although many children become liars because of feelings of insecurity, others do so without knowing it.

> *Your child might not know he's lying.*

A child who consumes large amounts of candy and junk food might have a low-blood-sugar condition that makes him legitimately blank out the fact that he's taken the sweet he craves. When a mother knows her child has eaten a cookie, asks him to confess, and hears him deny it, she calls him a liar. Confused as the child is, if he's called a liar often enough, he believes it and often becomes one.

If your child's little white lies are growing darker, eliminate sugars, refined starches, and junk food from his diet.

Increase these foods
   Brewer's yeast, wheat bran, cabbage, milk, eggs, roasted peanuts, the white meat of poultry, avocados, dates.

Suggested vitamins and minerals
   Vitamin B complex with niacin   50–100 mg. daily
   Children's multiple-vitamin-mineral supplement (1 daily)

129. The athlete

Athletic children are generally in pretty good physical shape to begin with, but they have to eat right to stay that way.

On the morning of a special athletic event, give your child a high-carbohydrate breakfast—whole-grain cereals or breads—but avoid foods loaded with sugar, honey, or corn syrup. (These tend to draw fluid into the gastrointestinal tract and can add to dehydration problems during endurance sports.)

Although an athletic child's actual protein requirement is no different from an ordinary child's, his expenditure of energy requires more calories, and his diet should have ample protein-rich foods and complete carbohydrates.

Include these foods (but not to excess)
Peas, beans, whole-grain cereals, pastas, breads, fresh fruits, meat, fish, eggs, milk, nuts, and soy products.

Suggested vitamins and minerals
Children's multiple-vitamin-mineral supplement with extra C and E (1 daily)

130. The diabetic child

A child with diabetes is unable to use sugars properly because of hormonal malfunction. Usually the child's insulin, which converts carbohydrates to glycogen, is insufficient to process the sugars, which then stay in the bloodstream and are excreted in the urine, depriving the brain and various organs of necessary energy. Artificial insulin must be given to correct the body's natural hormonal balance.

There are several forms of diabetes, but, in all, the foods that must be avoided are sugars and refined carbohydrates. (For hidden sugars in foods, see section 105.)

Brewer's yeast is good to include in the child's diet, but I'd advise checking with a nutritionally oriented pediatrician (see section 171) before adding it because three tablespoons have been known to reduce a child's need for insulin, and your child might need his dosage revised.

Suggested vitamins and minerals
Stress B complex   50–100 mg. daily
Vitamin C   500–1,000 mg. daily
Children's multiple-mineral supplement, with chromium (1 daily)

Be sure all supplements contain no added sugar or starch. (For a list of sugar-free liquid vitamins and medicines, see section 170.)

131. The forgetful child

The brain needs energy just as all the other parts of your child's body do, and if it doesn't have enough of the right energy, it cannot function properly. Glucose (blood sugar) is what the brain needs to function properly, and since glucose cannot be stored in the brain, it must be supplied regularly.

> *The wrong foods can make your child*
> *forget the right things.*

Low-blood sugar can cause blackouts and loss of memory; vitamin B$_6$ (pyridoxine) has been found to improve memory. Children who are lowering their blood-sugar levels with high intakes of sugars and refined starches, which require the B vitamins for metabolization, are doubly sabotaging their memories. These children are poor learners and are thought to be unintelligent, but they are often quite bright and merely victims of poor nutrition and an insufficient supply of pyridoxine.

Next time you're about to shout at your child for forgetting something, think about what he has—and has not—been eating.

Increase these foods
Nutritional yeast, liver, fresh vegetables, fish, eggs, beef, cabbage, wheat bran.

Suggested vitamins and minerals
Vitamin B complex   25–50 mg. daily
Choline   500–1,000 mg. daily

132. The restless sleeper

The best diet for a child who has trouble falling asleep or who tosses and turns nightly is one that includes ample amounts of tryptophan-rich foods, such as milk, bananas, turkey, and natural cheeses.

Suggested vitamins and minerals
Tryptophan   250–667 mg.
Vitamin B$_6$ 50–100 mg.
Magnesium   133 mg. chelated
All should be taken a half hour before bedtime with juice (no protein).

133. The hyperactive child

This child is one who has a poor attention span, is easily distracted, often has tantrums, and flits from one activity to another. Although bright, often he cannot retain information because of a chemical deficiency (usually norepinephrine) in his system; the chemical is needed for proper brain function. Drugs such as *Ritalin* and *Dexedrine* are often prescribed for such children, to compensate for the lack of norepinephrine; they usually have the effect of calming the child.

> *Allergies can be the cause.*

Much controversy abounds about hyperactivity. There are many theories for its cause—poor prenatal nutrition, brain damage at birth, chemical poisoning—but the current feeling is that a diet insufficient in B vitamins and high in refined carbohydrates, artificial colorings, and additives, and salicylate-containing foods may also be responsible.

Dr. Benjamin Feingold, founder of the Feingold Association of the United States (FAUS) specializing in the study of hyperactive children, has found that many children are hyperactive because of an allergy to aspirin and salicylate-containing foods, foods containing artificial colors and preservatives.

The largest use of salicylic acid is in the preparation of aspirin; another is in the preparation of synthetic oil of wintergreen. Salicylate is widely used as a flavoring agent in *candies, beverages, toothpastes, and powders*.

Salicylate is also used for enteric-coated pills (pills with a coating that protects them from absorption until they reach the intestine). Because phenylsalicylate absorbs ultraviolet light, it can be found, too, in antisunburn creams.

If your child is hyperactive, I advise that you keep him away from fluorescent lights and all refined carbohydrates and that you check labels for any foods containing salicylate. This is not to say that medication will then be unnecessary, but it's possible that in some cases it might be.

Increase these foods
Nutritional yeast, fish, beef, kelp, vegetables high in B vitamins.

Suggested vitamins and minerals
Vitamin B complex	25–50 mg. daily
Calcium	500 mg. daily
Magnesium	250 mg. daily

134. The slow learner

Children who have difficulty in retaining facts, catching on to new concepts, game rules, and so on, might be working under the extra handicap of a poor diet.

Much like the underachiever, the slow learner should eliminate refined foods and be put on a nutrition regimen high in B-complex vitamins. (See section 126, The Underachiever, for suggested diet and vitamins.)

135. The lazy child

Before you label a child lazy, look into his diet. Many children who sit around watching television are often too tired to do anything else. It's quite possible that your child avoids going to the store or taking out the garbage because he's actually too fatigued to do so.

Anemia is often the cause of what parents think of as laziness in children. A simple blood test can detect this condition, and iron supplements can correct it. (Mononucleosis—see section 161—can also be responsible.)

Increase these foods
Nutritional yeast, citrus fruits, leafy green and yellow vegetables, milk, meat, liver.

Suggested vitamins and minerals
Vitamin B complex	25–50 mg. daily
Vitamin C	100–1,000 mg. daily
Iron	10–15 mg. daily

136. The constipated child

A child who has hard, infrequent, and difficult passage of stools needs more roughage in his diet. (Keep in mind that it's not necessary for your child to have a bowel movement every twenty-four hours.) Sugar, white flour products, and refined foods all contribute to constipation and should be avoided.

Increase these foods
Raw vegetables and fruits; seeds and nuts for children over four.

Suggested vitamins and minerals
Acidophilus liquid*   1 tsp. 3 times daily
Vitamin C   100–500 mg. daily

* If stool becomes too loose, decrease dosage.

137. The child entering puberty

Puberty is a time when great hormonal changes are occurring in your child's body and when good nutrition is vital.

For girls, puberty begins with the onset of menstruation (menarche), which usually takes place sometime between the ages of nine and sixteen. Boys generally attain puberty later than girls, but thirteen is about average.

Because of the hormonal changes, there is often a high incidence of acne about this time, and foods rich in sugars, fats, salt, and refined carbohydrates can aggravate the condition.

Increase these foods
Leafy green and yellow vegetables, meat, fish, eggs, poultry, raw sunflower seeds, citrus fruits.

Suggested vitamins and minerals
Children's multiple-vitamin and mineral supplement (1 daily)
Stress B complex with vitamin C and zinc (1 daily)
Vitamin E, dry form, 100–200 IU daily

138. Any questions about chapter XIII?

My three-month-old daughter is very colicky and cries for hours at a time every night. Is there anything I can give her that might help?

The abdominal discomfort that your daughter has might be caused by a number of things—excessive gas, swallowed air, an allergy to her formula, or, if you're breast-feeding, something that you've eaten. Ordinary colic will usually disappear as the child's digestive system matures, but in the meanwhile sips of comfrey tea might help. Sometimes a potassium solution and a vitamin B complex (10–50 mg. daily) work wonders, but I'd advise checking with a nutritionally oriented pediatrician (see section 171) for the proper dosage for your child.

My son is eight and he's in pretty good health, except that he never has a simple cold—it always goes into a fever that keeps him out of school for three or four days. Is there some vitamin he's missing?

Not necessarily, but he could use some extra ones at the first sign of a sneeze. I'd suggest adding more citrus juices and fruits to his diet, along with fish and liver. And if you suspect he's coming down with something, I'd suggest you give him 1 tsp. of cod liver oil (a good source of vitamins A and D), a children's multiple-vitamin and mineral supplement, 100–1,000 mg. of vitamin C, and 100 mg. pantothenic acid daily to build up his resistance.

What can you suggest for a teething baby? My daughter is almost two years old, has only twelve teeth, and has come down with terrible colds cutting every one of them. The only thing I've been giving her is baby aspirin. Is there something better?

Definitely. The aspirin you're giving her is tripling her vitamin-C excretion at a time when she needs all her vitamins to build up her resistance. Teething doesn't cause colds; germs cause colds. But teething does lower a child's natural resistance. Unless your child is running a fever—an indication that infection has already set in—I'd suggest you concentrate on adding more citrus fruits and juices to her diet. Make sure she's getting enough vitamin-B-rich foods—and enough vitamin D.

Few natural foods contain ample amounts of vitamin D, not even milk, unless it's fortified. And the benefits of vitamin D on tooth formation can be expected only when the child's calcium and phosphorus intakes are satisfactory. Heredity plays a large part in how quickly a child's teeth erupt, but slow teething accompanied by illness seems to point to a nutrient deficiency. If your daughter is not taking supplementary vitamins, she ought to be. A consultation with a nutritionally oriented pediatrician (see section 171) might make life easier for both of you.

What could soothe the pressure caused by erupting teeth is letting her hold and gum a cold raw carrot. (It's a lot tastier than a teething ring.) And although your grandmother might suggest rubbing paregoric on the child's gums, I wouldn't. Paregoric is a narcotic and should not be given in any way, shape, or form to an infant unless you've been specifically directed to do so by a doctor.

Part Five

GETTING KIDS WELL SOONER

CHAPTER XIV

More Than an Ounce of Prevention

139. How to keep your child healthy

A parent has to become a black belt in the art of nutritional self-defense. What this means is that you have to recognize the enemies (all processed, refined, sugary, additive-filled, artificially flavored and colored foods) and keep them from your child, while supplying him with a variety of whole vitamin-rich foods at the same time. (See section 108.)

A good supplement regimen to help keep kids in all-around infection-fighting shape would be:

> A children's multiple-vitamin-mineral supplement, without artificial additives or sugar
> Vitamin B complex   50–100 mg.
> Vitamin C   100–1,000 mg.
> Vitamin E   100–200 IU
> Taken once or twice daily (depending on size, need, and age of child) with breakfast and dinner. (See section 71 for special situation cautions.)

140. Acne

The best way to help keep it away (or at least at bay) is to have your child avoid refined carbohydrates, fried foods, shellfish, and iodized salt and to eat plenty of plain yogurt.

The vitamin regimen I'd suggest for teenagers would be a multiple vitamin with 5,000 IU vitamin A; vitamin B complex (10–25 mg.); vitamin E, dry form (100–200 IU); and vitamin C (500–1,000 mg.), all once a day.

Flavored acidophilus liquid (1 tbsp.) three times daily.

141. Athlete's foot

A teenager who wears sneakers or runs barefoot all the time is a likely candidate for athlete's foot. Vitamin-C powder or crystals applied directly to the foot helps to eradicate this fungus infection. (The child's feet should be kept dry and out of shoes as much as possible until the infection clears.)

142. Bad breath

Your child might be brushing properly, but the problem might lie in his diet. Sometimes milk is the cause. Avoiding refined carbohydrates—which promote tooth decay—and adding foods rich in vitamins A, B, C, and niacin (see chapter II) to his menus can do a lot for eliminating "dragon breath."

Along with regular dental hygiene, you can try the child on 1 chlorophyll tablet or capsule daily; zinc (15 mg.) once or twice daily; acidophilus capsules (3) or flavored acidophilus (1 tbsp.) once or twice daily.

143. Burns

Put cold water on the burn immediately. To promote healing, have the child eat a diet that is high in protein and that includes fish liver oil, wheat germ, nutritional yeast, pumpkin and sunflower seeds, lamb chops, and nonfat dry milk. Also, plenty of fluids.

Vitamin C (up to 3,000 mg. daily, depending on severity of burn and age of child); vitamin B complex (50 mg.) three times a day; zinc (15 mg.) three times a day; vitamin A (10,000 IU) once or twice daily for a few days.

Vitamin E oil (28,000 IU) applied externally to the burn can help prevent scarring.

144. Broken bones

The healing of broken bones can be accelerated by adding more calcium and vitamin D to the child's diet. Foods such as milk, milk products, cheeses, salmon, peanuts, sunflower seeds, green vegetables, almonds, and apples all help.

For supplements, chelated calcium (500 mg.), chelated magnesium (250 mg.), and vitamin D (200–400 IU) can be taken daily for best results.

145. Canker sores

These usually appear after some sort of stress situation. A child with canker sores should avoid eating walnuts, chocolate, citrus fruits and juices, and he should increase his consumption of legumes, alfalfa sprouts, and plain (unsugared) yogurt.

Lysine (500 mg.) and vitamin C (500–1,000 mg.) taken daily; pantothenic acid (100 mg.) taken two to three times daily; acidophilus caps (3) taken one to three times daily, promote healing.

146. Cuts and bruises

Fresh citrus fruits and juices should be emphasized in the child's daily diet.

Vitamin C (500–1,000 mg.) with bioflavonoids, rutin, and hesperidin, taken once or twice daily, along with zinc (15 mg.) and vitamin E (100–200 IU) can help heal the "ouchies" faster.

147. Insect bites

Try to prevent them by having your child get enough thiamine (vitamin B_1). It's been found that vitamin B_1 creates a smell at the level of the skin that insects do not like. Foods rich in B_1 are brewer's yeast and liver. (See section 9 for others.)

If the child is stung, vitamin E oil or cream (20,000 IU to 28,000 IU) can be applied externally to relieve itch and sting.

148. Prickly heat

This common baby and children's rash usually occurs when hot weather begins. Tiny blisters often form on the clusters of minute pink pimples, and when they dry, they give the skin the appearance of a blotchy tan. An external application of 1 tsp. bicarbonate of soda mixed with 1 cup of water, patted on with cotton, helps.

Keep the child cool and dry and offer plenty of citrus juices and fruits. For infants, a vitamin-C supplement of 100–200 mg. daily can often bring relief. Older children can take 250–1,000 mg.

149. Poison oak and poison ivy

Contact with poison oak or ivy brings about clusters of small blisters of varying sizes on the child's skin. Vitamin E oil (28,000 IU) and aloe vera gel applied externally can alleviate some of the discomfort.

A child with poison ivy or poison oak should eat plenty of citrus fruits and juices, alfalfa sprouts, legumes (peas, beans), wheat germ, soy products, and fish liver oils. Vitamin C (100–500 mg.), preferably time-release, can be taken with breakfast and dinner.

Other supplements that have been shown to lessen the allergic reaction are vitamin E (100–400 IU) daily; vitamin B complex (25–50 mg.) with 100 mg. pantothenic acid taken one to three times daily; and vitamin A (5,000 IU) twice daily for five days a week.

150. Warts

They don't come from frogs, but that doesn't make them any more desirable. (They are suspected of being caused by viruses.) I'd advise adding soy products, wheat germ, fish liver oils, and brewer's yeast to your child's diet as both a preventive measure and a healing one.

Vitamin E oil (28,000 IU) applied externally one to three times daily has been found to help clear up warts.

As a supplement, vitamin E (100–200 IU) and vitamin C (500–1,000 mg.) can be taken daily, along with vitamin A (10,000 IU)—which should be taken only five days a week and omitted for two—and zinc (15 mg.).

151. Any questions about chapter XIV?

My twelve-year-old daughter bites her fingernails and hates herself for doing it but can't seem to stop. Does this indicate a vitamin deficiency, or is it just nervousness? Are there any remedies?

Nail biting is generally an indication of some sort of anxiety or tenseness. A vitamin B complex that includes vitamin C and zinc can help. Also, calcium, magnesium, and inositol are the best relaxants I know (one chelated calcium and magnesium tablet two times daily). You can try giving her tryptophan at bedtime (500 mg. taken with juice), which can help her sleep better and make her feel less anxious during the day.

As an immediate remedy, ask your pharmacist for some oil of mustard and paint it on her fingernails; the taste will deter her from biting.

My teenage daughter gets terrible cramps during menstruation; and a week before her period, she starts gaining waterweight, which doesn't disappear until almost two weeks later. Would dietary changes help either of these problems?

There's a very good chance of it. Vitamin B_6 (pyridoxine) is a natural diuretic and also reduces muscle spasms, which means it can help alleviate her cramps as well as the bloating. Liver, brewer's yeast, wheat germ, and cantaloupe are good sources of vitamin B_6 and should be emphasized in her diet. A cantaloupe shake (1 cup milk, ¼ cantaloupe, 1 tsp. honey, 1 tsp. protein powder, blended with 3 ice cubes) is a delicious naturally diuretic drink. Adding supplements of vitamin B_6 (50 mg.) twice daily, along with a vitamin B complex, will probably bring relief even faster.

Are there any vitamins that can help a child who has dandruff?

There are some that might help. I'd suggest increasing vitamin-B-rich foods in the diet and supplementing with a B-complex (50–100 mg.) that includes vitamin C and zinc, along with vitamin E (100–200 IU) daily, and vitamin A (5,000–10,000 IU) with breakfast five days a week. Selenium-rich yeast (1 tsp.) mixed in milk or juice can also be beneficial. A daily jojoba oil scalp massage and shampoo can often squelch the "snowstorm."

CHAPTER XV

Common Childhood Diseases

152. The importance of nutrition during illness

A child who is sick is under stress. Adrenal glands deprived of nutrients cannot function properly, and the child's usual rough-and-ready stress-fighting team of vitamins C, B_6, folic acid, and pantothenic acid becomes sorely handicapped.

Children require these vitamins to effectively use all the other nutrients that keep them healthy, happy, and growing; therefore, it's even more important that they are well supplied with them when illness and fever take their nutritional toll.

Again, these food and supplement regimens are not intended as medical advice, but as a guide to working with your child's doctor, who'll know if any foods are contraindicated while the child is on prescribed medication. (See section 168.)

153. Bronchitis

A child with bronchitis has an inflammation of his bronchial-tube lining and needs plenty of vitamin-B-rich foods to counteract the stress of the disease on his body.

Wheat germ should be sprinkled liberally on whatever the child eats. Citrus fruits and juices should be increased. Soybeans and fish liver oils are also nutrient-filled pluses for the diet.

Blender nutrient bonus: Blend 1 cup cantaloupe, ½ cup orange juice, juice of ½ lemon, and ice.

My supplement suggestions
    Vitamin A (10,000 IU) daily for 5 days a week
    Vitamin C (500 mg.), time-release, taken with breakfast
      and dinner

Vitamin E (100-200 IU), dry form, once or twice daily
Acidophilus (3 caps or 1 tbsp. flavored) daily
Six to eight glasses water daily

154. Chicken pox

The fever and itching that accompany this stock childhood disease, which is caused by a virus closely related to that of shingles, can deplete a child of many nutrients. Citrus fruits and juices should be increased (if possible), and wheat germ and soybean products should be included in the child's daily food intake.

Blender nutrient bonus: Blend ½ cup each of strawberries, low-fat yogurt, and ice cubes.

My supplement suggestions
>   Rose hips vitamin C (500 mg.), time-release, taken with breakfast and dinner
>   Vitamin E (100–200 IU) once or twice daily for five days a week until sores heal
>   Children's multivitamin and mineral supplement twice daily with food

155. Colitis

This upsetting illness of alternating diarrhea and constipation, as well as abdominal pain, is often triggered by emotional upset. Diet is of prime importance. Check with a nutritionally oriented pediatrician (see section 171) so that you can properly evaluate your child's condition.

Latest treatments include and recommend bran, bulk and fiber foods, along with yogurt, bananas, and potatoes (real, not instant).

Blender nutrient bonus: Blend ½ banana, ½ cup yogurt, and ice cubes.

My supplement suggestions
>   Children's multiple-vitamin and mineral supplement, 1 daily
>   Potassium (99 mg.), 1 daily
>   Sugarless cabbage juice (vitamin U), 1 glass three times daily

Acidophilus (3 caps or 1 tbsp. liquid), twice daily
Bran (1 tbsp. or 3–6 tablets) daily

156. Eye infections

Pinkeye (which can be caused by strepto-, staphylo-, and
pneumococcus, as well as influenza bacillus) is only one of
several types of conjunctivitis that kids contract, and conjunctivitis is only one of the many types of eye infections.

If your child has an eye infection, good additions to his
diet would be citrus fruits or juices, nutritional yeast, oatmeal, liver, carrots, milk, and fish liver oils.

Blender nutrient bonus: Blend 1½ cups pineapple juice, 1
large carrot (cut up), and ½ cup ice cubes.

My supplement suggestions
Vitamin A (5,000–10,000 IU) daily for five days a week
Vitamin B complex with C, time-release, with breakfast
and dinner daily
Vitamin E (100 IU), dry form, with breakfast and dinner
daily

157. Hypoglycemia

This low-blood-sugar condition presents a situation much
like diabetes, wherein the child's body is unable to metabolize carbohydrates normally. Because a hypoglycemic child's
system essentially overreacts to sugar, producing too much
insulin, the key to raising the blood-sugar levels is *not* by
feeding the child more rapidly metabolized carbohydrates but
by offering more protein. (See section 55.)

It's a good idea to have the child eat smaller meals more
often—every two or three hours—to keep blood-sugar levels
up.

Blender nutrient bonus: Blend 1 cup unsweetened pineapple juice, 1 banana, 1 tbsp. milk-and-egg protein powder, and
2–3 ice cubes.

My supplement suggestions
Children's multiple-vitamin and mineral supplement
Vitamin C (100–500 mg.), time-release

Vitamin E (100–200 IU), dry form
Pantothenic acid (50–100 mg.)
All taken with breakfast and dinner daily

158. Impetigo

Children often contract this infection, which is caused by staphylococcus or streptococcus germs, by scratching and infecting insect bites, thereby allowing the germs to invade the broken skin. Because the child's body is being stressed by this germ invasion, it's advisable to emphasize foods rich in vitamins B complex, A, C, and D. Wheat germ, fish liver oils, soybean products, and citrus fruits are particularly good. So are milk and peanuts.

Blender nutrient bonus: Blend 1 cup nonfat milk, ¼ tsp. cinnamon, ¼ cup peanut butter, 1–3 tsp. molasses, 2–3 ice cubes.

My supplement suggestions
Vitamin A (5,000 IU) and Vitamin D (200 IU) daily for four to five days a week
Vitamin E (100–200 IU) daily
Rose hips vitamin C (100–500 mg.) with breakfast and dinner daily

159. Influenza (Flu)

Every year thousands of children come down with the flu.

Since there are many different strains of influenza viruses, even if your child has an immunity to one— because he was down with it last year—doesn't mean that he'll be immune to the one going around this year. Influenza is highly contagious and spreads rapidly in schools.

Antibiotics and sulfa drugs are ineffective against the influenza virus, but because secondary infections often develop, many doctors prescribe them right from the onset, causing even more vitamins to be depleted from the child's already stressed system. (See section 169.)

The best protection for your child is a good diet and to keep him away from crowds as much as possible during the flu season.

If your child does come down with the flu, keep his fighting forces going with foods that contain the important B and C vitamins. Your child's appetite might not be up to par, so try camouflaged nutrition. (See section 55.)

Blender nutrient bonus: Blend ¾ cup dry nonfat milk, ½ tsp. vanilla, 1 cup fresh or frozen berries (without sugar), ½ cup water, and 4–6 ice cubes.

My supplement suggestions
   Children's multivitamin and mineral supplement and vitamin C (100–1,000 mg.) taken daily with breakfast and dinner
   Vitamin E (100–200 IU) daily
   Vitamin B complex (50–100 mg.) daily

160. Measles

There is now a preventive vaccine for measles, but the virus (which is one of the most contagious) still manages to snare a large number of unprotected children each year. For some children, the disease is nothing more than a mild rash and low fever; for others, it is quite severe and accompanied by a heavy cough. Your child's body needs the right foods and vitamins to fight and recover from this one.

Plenty of milk, eggs, carrots, and green vegetables are helpful, as are citrus fruits and juices, wheat germ, and soybean products.

Blender nutrient bonus: Blend ¾ cup pineapple juice, ½ cup orange juice, ¼ cup nonfat dry milk, ¼ cup blanched almonds, and ½ cup ice.

My suggested supplements
   Vitamin A (5,000 IU) one to two times daily for four to five days a week
   Rose hips vitamin C (100–500 mg.) with breakfast and dinner
   Vitamin E (100–400 IU) daily

161. Mononucleosis

Young adolescents seem to be particularly susceptible to mono (glandular fever), or "the kissing disease" as it's often called, but young children are not immune. Characterized by fatigue and often a sore throat that won't respond to antibiotics, this disease is not always detected by ordinary blood tests and sometimes requires a special "mono" blood test.

Recuperation from mono requires a diet high in vitamin C and all the B vitamins. To help a child on the mend, add alfalfa sprouts to salads, sprinkle wheat germ over yogurt, and offer bananas and citrus fruits and juices often.

Blender nutrient bonus: Blend ½ cup each tomato juice, buttermilk, and yogurt. Chill.

My suggested supplements
    Children's multiple-vitamin and mineral supplement
    Rose hips vitamin C (100–500 mg.)
    Vitamin B complex (50 mg.)
    All taken with breakfast and dinner daily
    Potassium (99 mg.) 1 daily

162. Mumps

There is a vaccine to prevent mumps, but the disease is still common among children and nutritionally it is quite debilitating. The virus is not restricted to the salivary glands and is capable of spreading throughout the child's entire system.

In planning the child's diet, go heavy on the citrus juices and try to include wheat germ and soybean products.

Blender nutrient bonus: Blend 1 cup of milk, ¼ of a fresh cantaloupe, 1 tsp. honey, 1 tbsp. milk-and-egg protein powder, and 3 ice cubes.

My suggested supplements
    Vitamin A (5,000 IU) with breakfast and dinner five
       days during week of illness
    Rose hips vitamin C (100–500 mg.) daily with breakfast
       and dinner
    Vitamin E (100–200 IU) daily

163. Tonsillitis

"My throat hurts" is one of the most common complaints of illness among children, and tonsillitis—an inflammation of the tonsils—is one of the most common childhood diseases.

A child who's been on a nutritional self-defense diet is more likely to resist the disease and to recover from it.

Citrus fruits and juices, plain yogurt, and protein-rich broths are better than get-well cards for a speedy recovery.

Blender nutrient bonus: Blend equal amounts of grapefruit and cranberry juice, then stir in a tablespoon of lowfat yogurt.

> *My suggested supplements*
> Children's multiple-vitamin and mineral supplement (that includes at least 5,000 IU vitamin A) daily
> Rose hips vitamin C (100–500 mg.) with breakfast and dinner
> Acidophilus (3 caps) one to three times daily
> Six glasses of water daily

164. Stomachaches

When a child gets a stomachache, it could signal the onset of an illness as well as an upcoming history test. Take all stomachaches seriously, and consult your doctor if there's real discomfort involved.

As a suggestion, have your child eat more slowly and drink liquids (neither too hot nor too cold) a half hour before or after meals. A deficiency of niacin can decrease hydrochloric acid (HCL) and cause aches.

A distressed stomach doesn't want food, and it's best to let it have its way for a while. Herb tea might help.

> *My suggested supplements (to be used preventively, not while the child has the stomachache)*
> Vitamin B complex (25–50 mg.) daily
> Pantothenic acid (50–100 mg.) one to two times daily
> Chewable papaya enzymes, 1–2 after meals

165. Any questions about chapter XV?

My son comes down with the same strep throat at least twice a year. Is there some way I can build up his immunity?

I doubt if he comes down with the *same* streptococcus infection, since immunity follows each strep throat. But there are many different strains of streptococci that do produce the same illness. I'd suspect his resistance to infection is low and that a major overhauling of his diet is in order.

He should be eating foods high in vitamin A—carrots, spinach, liver, eggs, dairy products—which promote such resistance. Also, plenty of vitamin-C-filled citrus fruits and juices and lots of whole grains, nuts, and yeast to replenish his depleted B vitamins. I'd suggest supplementing this diet with a good children's multivitamin and mineral supplement twice daily; vitamin C (100–500 mg.), three times daily; and a B complex with ample folic acid, two—even three times a day.

Do you believe in "feeding a cold" and "starving a fever"?

I believe in feeding a cold with vitamin C—at every meal and in every way. Vitamin C is not just in orange juice (see section 17); and whole meals can be doubled in C content with a little forethought. As for "starving a fever," not quite. A child with fever eats little, but what he does should count. If he'll sip juice, add vitamin C liquid or powder to it so that a little can do a lot. If you can get him to drink some soup or broth, make sure it's made from good nutrient-rich stock. Heavy meals are not in order and fluids are essential, so offer high-protein shakes or popsicles (see section 55) several times a day. A children's multiple-vitamin and mineral supplement, B complex (50 mg.), and vitamin C (100–500 mg.) should be taken twice daily. Vitamin A (5,000 IU) can be taken twice daily for four to five days a week while the child is ill.

CHAPTER XVI

Children's Medicines

166. Medicines vs. vitamins—the big battle

Medicines can do wonderful things for kids. If prescribed and taken correctly, they can cure a variety of illnesses that could not be combatted any other way. But far too often they are prescribed unnecessarily, simply because the medical establishment refuses to recognize the curative and preventive power of vitamins and natural foods.

> *Does your child really need that Rx?*

Many doctors feel threatened by the overwhelming evidence that there are vitamins that can do the work of drugs. Vitamins are natural substances and therefore are not under government or the doctor's control. The giant drug corporations aren't pleased with vitamins either, because they can't be patented; which means the drug corporations can't make money from them.

Orthomolecular and nutritionally oriented physicians, on the other hand, are trying vitamin and natural-food regimens before resorting to drugs—and having remarkable success. Dr. Robert C. Atkins, author of *Dr. Atkins' Diet Revolution,* has taken patients off dangerous barbiturates and put them on natural regimens of inositol and pantothenic acid that have been equally effective.

Dr. Richard Swenski of Glen Lyon, Pennsylvania, has successfully treated young patients with alfalfa (which contains vitamins A, E, K, B, D, iron, potassium, phosphorus, chlorine, sodium, silicon, and magnesium, in addition to eight enzymes critical for food assimilation) for numerous illnesses that had previously been unsuccessfully treated with drugs.

167. Vitamins that can work as medicines

Before popping a synthetic antibiotic into your child's mouth at the first sniffle, why not take a good look around nature's pharmacy?

- Onions, garlic, radishes, and leeks all contain a natural antibiotic called *allicin*. Unlike prescription antibiotics, allicin can destroy disease germs without sweeping away the friendly bacteria in doing so. (You can use these vegetables in soups, salads, meat loaves, even the child's favorite spaghetti sauce.)
- A small slice of fresh ginger root, sucked on two or three times a day, is a natural sore-throat preventive. Also, an effective natural gargle is a tea made from goldenseal root and gum myrrh (herbs that can be found in health food stores). These herbs contain natural antibacterial and antiseptic properties.
- A natural diuretic is cranberry juice, which has also been found effective in staving off a variety of infectious diseases. (You can freeze the cranberry juice in an ice cube tray, add popsicle sticks when partly frozen, and your kids will have a refreshing snack!)
- All jokes aside, chicken soup (homemade) really has antihistamine properties and can work wonders for children's colds.
- Commercial laxatives can be avoided by adding more bran to your child's diet. (Popcorn is a fine source of roughage!)
- Before asking a doctor for tranquilizers for your nervous child, try adding more vitamin-B-rich foods to his diet, along with a stress B-complex supplement with vitamin C (two to three times a day).
- Instead of dosing your child with *Tums, Rolaids,* or *Alka-Seltzer* for heartburn, try giving him a multiple digestive enzyme.

168. Mixing medicines and foods

Keeping your child on a nutritious diet is important when he's ill, but if the child is on medication, there are certain foods that might interact adversely with the medicine or be necessary for its effectiveness, and you should be aware of them.

Medicine (trade name)	Foods to Watch
Acetaminophen (*Tylenol, Datril, Nebs, Tempra, Valadol*)	Carbohydrates, such as crackers or jellies, may slow the medicine's absorption rate and increase the time it takes to be effective.
Ampicillin (*Amcill, Polycillin, Omnipen, Penbritin, Principen*)	Should be administered on an empty stomach—thirty minutes before giving food. Sugars, soft drinks, and citrus juices, when taken with the medicine, decrease its antibacterial action.
Demeclocycline (*Declomycin*)	Milk and dairy products and foods high in iron inhibit the absorption of this tetracycline and shouldn't be taken at the same time.
Erythromycin (*E-Mycin, Ilosone, Pediamycin, Erythrocin, Robimycin*)	Sugars, soft drinks, and citrus fruit juices promote rapid breakdown of drug in the stomach and decrease the medicine's antibacterial action.
Griseofulvin (*Fulvicin, Grifulvin V, Grisactin*)	This antifungal medication is most effective when taken with meals high in fat content (margarine, butter, pork, and so on).
Iron (*Feosol, Fergon,* other iron-fortified preparations)	Milk, eggs, cereals, and dairy products in general should not be taken with iron medications because these foods inhibit the iron's absorption.

Medicine (trade name)	*Foods to Watch*
Methenamine Mandelate (*Mandelamine*)	An acidic urine is required for effectiveness, so increase vitamin-C-rich fruits and juices. Do not give child carbonated beverages.
Penicillin (*Penicillin G, Penn-Vee K, V-Cillin K, Compocillin-V, Compocillin-VK, Pentids*)	Same as for ampicillin.
Phenobarbital (*Luminal*)	Avoid giving medication with cocoa, chocolate, and sodas containing caffeine.
Phenytoin (*Dilantin, Di-Len, Diphen, Diphentoin, Di-Phenylhydantoin*)	Keep child away from foods containing MSG. This drug increases the absorption rate of MSG, which can cause general weakness and numbness.
Tetracycline (*Achromycin V, Cyclopar, Panmycin, Robitet, Sumycin, Tetracyn*)	Same as for demeclocycline.
Thyroid (*Proloid, Synthroid*)	Avoid giving child cabbage, carrots, kale, cauliflower, peaches, pears, spinach, Brussels sprouts, and turnips while he's on medication, since these foods will further inhibit thyroid hormone activity and interfere with the medicine.
Warfarin (*Coumadin, Panwarfin*)	Foods such as leafy vegetables, especially spinach, cauliflower, and Brussels sprouts, as well as potatoes, should be avoided because they are high in vitamin K and will decrease the medicine's effectiveness.

169. Medicines that deplete vitamins

ASPIRIN
(and all products containing aspirin, such as Aspergum, Alka-Seltzer, Congespirin)

Aspirin can triple the rate of excretion of your child's vitamin C. It also depletes the child of essential B_1 (thiamine) and folic acid. It's important to replace these vitamins in your child's diet by supplying ample amounts of citrus fruits and juices, nutritional yeast, leafy green vegetables, and other foods high in B vitamins.

A vitamin B-complex with C is recommended as a supplement.

CHILDREN'S COUGH SYRUPS
(if they contain alcohol)

Alcohol-containing cough syrups can drain your child of B vitamins, especially folic acid, and vitamin B_{12}. The syrups also deplete iron, magnesium, and zinc. While your child is on medication, increase the amount of vitamin-B-rich foods in his diet, as well as nuts, apples, eggs, nonfat dry milk, and meat.

A children's multiple-vitamin mineral supplement, vitamin C (100–500 mg.) daily, and vitamin A (5,000 IU) five days a week, while the child is on medication, is recommended as a supplement.

ANTACIDS
(Maalox and other preparations that combine aluminum and magnesium hydroxides)

A child taking Maalox is being unknowingly depleted of vitamin A and vitamin B_1. This medicine, and other antacids containing the combination of aluminum and magnesium hydroxides, also decrease the child's absorption of iron and phosphate.

Fish liver oils, yogurt, and nutritional yeast are advisable additions to a child's diet if he's taking Maalox. (Acidic foods should be avoided.)

Acidophilus (3 caps or 1 tbsp. flavored) is suggested as a supplement one to three times daily, along with papaya enzymes.

MILK OF MAGNESIA
    Same as antacids.

MINERAL OIL
    Long-term use of mineral oil can decrease vitamin A and carotene absorption to the point where signs of deficiency appear. Also depleted are vitamins D, E, and K; calcium and phosphates are decreased in absorption, as is vitamin C. Bulk and fiber foods should be added to the child's diet.
    A supplement of vitamin A (5,000 IU), water-soluble, is recommended. It should be given daily, five days a week, several hours before taking mineral oil.
    I strongly suggest you *do not* give your child mineral oil unless you have been specifically directed to do so by a physician.

PENICILLIN PRODUCTS
(including all ampicillin products)
    The big depletion with these antibiotics is potassium. Foods high in potassium, such as bananas, potatoes (with skin), and all citrus fruits, tomatoes, sunflower seeds, and yogurt, should be dispensed freely to the child during treatment.
    A children's multiple-vitamin and mineral supplement, vitamin C (500–1,000 mg.), a stress B complex, and zinc (15 mg.) are recommended as daily supplements.

PHENOBARBITAL (*Luminal*)
    This medication takes its toll on children by depriving them of some of the vitamins they obviously need most, such as folic acid and vitamin B_{12}, as well as vitamin D and vitamin K.
    Menus that include tuna, milk, salmon, cantaloupe, eggs, deep-green leafy vegetables, and alfalfa can help.
    A vitamin B-complex supplement including niacinamide and magnesium is recommended as a supplement while the child is on the medication.

SULFONAMIDES
    These sulfa medications are usually prescribed for urinary tract infections and are known depleters of vitamin K.
    Use safflower oil for cooking the child's meals and include plenty of yogurt, egg yolks, leafy greens, and alfalfa in his meals. And keep the child out of direct sunlight while he is taking the medicine.

TETRACYCLINES
(the entire family—including all the "-mycins")

The medicine goes down, but the vitamins and minerals do also: vitamin K, calcium, magnesium, iron, zinc, vitamin C, vitamin B_2, folic acid, and niacin are all casualties.

Children on tetracycline antibiotics should have their diets laced with iron-rich foods—meat, farina, dried peaches, nuts, asparagus, oatmeal—and those high in calcium (see section 32).

Supplements of vitamin C (100–500 mg.), vitamin B complex (25–50 mg.), and acidophilus (3 caps or 1 tbsp. liquid) are suggested for every day that the child is taking the medicine.

170. Your child doesn't need sugar to get well

All too often, the Rx and over-the-counter liquid preparations that are prescribed for children are loaded with sugar. But sugar-free medicines are available and, in most cases, will be substituted on request by your doctor or pharmacist for a particular medicine's sugary twin.

SUGAR-FREE MEDICINES

Antacids and Digestants

Aludrox	Milk of Bismuth
Aluscop	Mylanta Liquid
Camalox	Mylanta-II Liquid
Creamalin	Mylicon Drops
Delcid	Pepto-Bismol
Digestamic	Probilagol
Dimacid Gel	Riopan Suspension
Estomul-M	Robalate Elixir
Gelusil (Plain, Flavor Pack)	Taka-Diastase
Kolantyl	Titralac
Maalox Suspension	Trisogel
	WinGel

Antiasthmatics and Bronchodilators

Alupent Syrup	Neothylline Elixir
Co-Xan	Neothylline-G Elixir

SUGAR-FREE MEDICINES

Antiasthmatics and Bronchodilators

Elixophyllin
Ephed-Organidin Elixir
Isuprel Compound Elixir
Lixaminol
Metaprel Syrup
Mudrane GG

Synophylate
Tedral Elixir
Tedral Pediatric Suspension
Theo-Organidin
Theophylline Elixir

Antibiotics and Anti-infectives

Antiminth Suspension
Compocillin-V Oral
  Suspension
Furadantin Oral
  Suspension
Furoxone Liquid
Mandelamine Suspension
NegGram Suspension
Robitet Suspension

Tao Oral Suspension
Terramycin Drops
Terramycin Syrup
Tetrachel-S Syrup, Pediatric
  Drops
Tetracyn Syrup
Thiosulfil Suspension
Vibramycin Syrup

Anticonvulsants

Mysoline Suspension

Antidepressants and Stimulants

Aventyl Liquid
Cenalene

Coramine Oral Solution
Sinequan Oral Concentrate

Antidiarrheals

Butibel-Gel
Coly-Mycin Pediatric
  Suspension
Corrective Mixture
Corrective Mixture
  w/Paregoric
Furoxone Suspension
Infantol
Infantol Pink
Kaolin-Mixture w/Pectin
  N.F.
Kaolin-Pectin Suspension

Kaolin-Pectin w/Neomycin
Kaopectate
Kaopectate Concentrate
    Anti-diarrhea Medicine
Lomotil
Opium Tincture
Paregoric (Parke-Davis)
Parepectolin
Pargel (Parke-Davis)
Pecto-Kalin
Quintess

SUGAR-FREE MEDICINES

Antispasmodics

Belladonna Alkaloids
w/Pb Elixir

Belladonna Tincture
(Parke-Davis)

Cough and Cold Preparations

Cerose
Cerose-DM
Cetro-Cirose
Cidicol
Clistin Expectorant
Colrex Compound Elixir
Colrex Expectorant
Colrex Syrup
Conar
Coryban-D Syrup
Covanamine Liquid
Covangesic Liquid
Co-Xan
Dimetapp Elixir
Hycomine Pediatric Syrup
Hycomine Syrup
Isoclor Liquid

Lanatuss
Organidin Solution
Ornacol Liquid
Orrini-Tuss
Prunicodeine
Romilar III, Syrup
Ryna-C Syrup
Sorbutuss
Spantuss
Terpin Hydrate & Codeine
(Parke-Davis)
Tussar SF
Tussionex Suspension
Tussi-Organidin
Tussi-Organidin DM
Tuss-Ornade

Laxatives and Stool Softeners

Agoral (Plain and
Flavored)
Cascara Sagrada F.E.
Aromatic #689 (Parke-
Davis)
Castor Oil
Castor Oil (Flavored)
Colace Liquid
Cologel
Haley's M-O
Kondremul, Plain/
Phenolphthalein and
w/Cascara
Magnesia-Alumina Oral
Suspension

Milk of Bismuth
(Parke-Davis)
Milk of Magnesia
(Parke-Davis)
Milk of Magnesia-Cascara
Suspension
Milk of Magnesia-Mineral
Oil Emulsion
Mineral Oil (Parke-
Davis)
Mint-O-Mag
Neoloid
Peri-Colace
Phospho-Soda
Rectalad

SUGAR-FREE MEDICINES

Miscellaneous

Cēpacol
Chloraseptic
Decadron Elixir
Glycerin Solution
  (Flavored) 50 percent
Kaochlor Concentrate
Kaochlor S-F
Kaon Elixir
Kay Ciel Elixir

Kolyum
Paradione Solution
PfiKlor
Potassium Chloride Liquid
Potassium Chloride Powder
Potassium Gluconate Elixir
Potassium Iodide Liquid
Potassium Triplex
Tylenol Drops

Sedatives, Tranquilizers

Amytal Elixir
Butisol Sodium Elixir
Haldol Concentrate
Mellaril Concentrate
  30 mg/ml
Permitil Oral Concentrate
Phenobarbital Liquid 100
  mg/5ml.

Sedadrops
Serentil Concentrate
Thorazine Concentrate
Triclos Liquid
Vesprin Suspension
Vistaril Suspension

Vitamins, Minerals, Lipotropics

Adelflor Drops
Aquasol A Drops
Aquasol E Drops
Betalin Complex Elixir
C-B Time
Cecon Solution
Ce-Vi-Sol Drops
Cod Liver Oil
Drisdol in Propylene
  Glycol
Ferrolip Syrup
Iberet-Liquid Oral Solution
Kaochlor S-F Ten Percent
  Liquid
Karidum

Niferex Elixir
Novacebrin Drops
Novacebrin w/Fluoride
  Drops
Pediaflor
PfiKlor
Phos-Flur Oral Rinse
Poly-Vi-Flor Drops
Poly-Vi-Sol Drops
Poly-Vi-Sol w/Iron Drops
Potassium Chloride
Potassium Gluconate
Potassium Triplex
Super D Oil
Theragran Liquid

SUGAR-FREE MEDICINES

Vitamins, Minerals, Lipotropics

Kay Ciel
Lipomul-Oral
Lipotriad
Liqui-Cee
Luride Drops

Toleron Suspension
Tri-Vi-Flor Drops
Tri-Vi-Sol w/Iron Drops
Vi-Daylin/F ADC Drops
Vi-Sorbin

171. Where to find a nutritionally oriented pediatrician

International College of Applied Nutrition
Box 386
La Habra, California 90631

International Academy of Preventative Medicine
10409 Town and Country Way, Suite 200
Houston, Texas 77024

Orthomolecular Medicine Society
2698 Pacific Avenue
San Francisco, California 94115

American Academy of Medical Preventics
2811 L Street, Suite 205
Sacramento, California 95816

International Academy of Metabology, Inc.
P.O. Box 15157
Las Cruces, New Mexico 88001

172. Any questions about chapter XVI?

Last summer, when my sixteen-year-old son was taking Declomycin, he was told not to go to the beach while on the medication. I thought sunlight provided vitamins. Why was he told not to go?

Declomycin, even more than other tetracycline medications, sensitizes the skin to sunlight. A long day at the beach could have resulted in a severe sunburn.

I've tried to give my daughter, aged eight, Pepto-Bismol to calm her stomach, which gets queasy when she's on antibiot-

ics. But she hates it and just gets more upset when I force it down. Is there any natural remedy that might help?

Yes, there is. But first you should know that Pepto-Bismol, or any other antacid, is the wrong thing to give a child if the antibiotic she's on is a tetracycline. The ingredients in antacids block the absorption of the drug, inhibiting its effectiveness. I'd recommend giving your daughter a cup of spearmint tea. It should settle her stomach nicely and alleviate any nausea. (Peppermint tea works, too, but the spearmint is milder and usually easier for the child to take.)

My two sons had the identical fungus infection, and both received the same drug, Fulvicin. The medicine worked very quickly for my older son (who's heavy), but not for my younger one (who's quite thin). Have you any idea why?

There could be numerous reasons, all best discussed with your physician. But your sons obviously have different eating habits, and that might be the key. Fulvicin works best when taken in conjunction with high-fat diets. If your older son was eating fats and your younger son was not, that might explain it.

Afterword

It is my hope that this book has enabled you to see the inestimable value of good nutrition for your children and has offered you enough flexible guidelines to implement practical programs that you can work in your own household for your own kids.

Don't be discouraged if your new nutritional enlightenment is not greeted with immediate enthusiasm by the younger members of your family. Kids are notorious creatures of habits (not necessarily good ones), and changing their eating patterns takes time and patience. But the rewards are worth it. Making your children aware of these rewards, explaining what's-in-it-for-them, is not only helpful but essential preparation for the time when they're old enough to make their own food decisions for themselves and for their kids.

My aim has been to create a book that could serve as a handy nutrition counselor, one that could be called upon from time to time to suggest recipes, regimens, and references for different situations as they arise—essentially, a book that could grow with your children and their needs for vitamins, which I firmly believe are as important as love. I hope that I've succeeded, and that the evidence of this success will be the continuing vitality and happiness of your children in the years ahead.

EARL L. MINDELL, R.Ph., Ph.D.

Los Angeles
April 5, 1981

Glossary

Absorption: the process by which nutrients are passed into the bloodstream.

Acetate: a derivative of acetic acid.

Acetic acid: used as a synthetic flavoring agent, one of the first food additives (vinegar is approximately 4 to 6 percent acetic acid); it is found naturally in cheese, coffee, grapes, peaches, raspberries, and strawberries; Generally Recognized As Safe (GRAS) when used only in packaging.

Acetone: a colorless solvent for fat, oils, and waxes, which is obtained by fermentation (inhalation can irritate lungs, and large amounts have a narcotic effect).

Acid: a water-soluble substance with sour taste.

Adrenals: the glands, located above each kidney, that manufacture adrenaline.

Alkali: an acid-neutralizing substance (sodium bicarbonate is an alkali used for excess acidity in foods).

Allergen: a substance that causes an allergy.

Alzheimer's disease: a progressively degenerative disease, involved with loss of memory, which new research indicates might be helped with extra choline.

Amino acid chelates: chelated minerals that have been produced by many of the same processes nature uses to chelate minerals in the body; in the digestive tract, nature surrounds the elemental minerals with amino acid, permitting them to be absorbed into the bloodstream.

Amino acids: the organic compounds from which proteins are constructed; there are twenty-two known amino acids, but only nine are indispensable nutrients for man—histidine, isoleucine, leucine, lysine, total S-containing amino acids, total aromatic amino acids, threonine, tryptophan, and valine.

Anorexia: loss of appetite.

Antibiotic: any of various substances that are effective in inhibiting or destroying bacteria.

Anticoagulant: something that delays or prevents blood-clotting.

Antigen: any substance not normally present in the body that stimulates the body to produce antibodies.

Antihistamine: a drug used to reduce effects associated with histamine production in allergies and colds.

Antioxidant: a substance that can protect another substance from oxidation; added to foods to keep oxygen from changing the food's color.

Antitoxin: an antibody formed in response to, and capable of neutralizing, a poison of biologic origin.

Assimilation: the process whereby nutrients are used by the body and changed into living tissue.

Ataxia: loss of coordinated movement caused by disease of nervous system.

ATP: a molecule called adenosine triphosphate, the fuel of life, a nucleotide—building block of nucleic acid—that produces biological energy with B_1, B_2, B_3, and pantothenic acid.

Avidin: a protein in egg white capable of inactivating biotin.

Bariatrician: a weight-control doctor.

BHA: butylated hydroxyanisole; a preservative and antioxidant used in many products; insoluble in water; can be toxic to the kidneys.

BHT: butylated hydroxytoluene; a solid, white crystalline antioxidant used to retard spoilage of many foods; can be more toxic to the kidney than its nearly identical chemical cousin BHA.

Bioflavonoids: usually from orange and lemon rinds, these citrus-flavored compounds needed to maintain healthy blood-vessel walls are widely available in plants, citrus fruits, and rose hips; known as vitamin P complex.

Calciferol: a colorless, odorless crystalline material, insoluble in water; soluble in fats; a synthetic form of vitamin D made by irradiating ergosterol with ultraviolet light.

Calcium gluconate: an organic form of calcium.

Capillary: a minute blood vessel, one of many that connect the arteries and veins.

Carcinogen: a cancer-causing substance.

Carotene: an orange-yellow pigment occurring in many plants and capable of being converted into vitamin A in the body.

Casein: the protein in milk that has become the standard by which protein quality is measured.

Catabolism: the metabolic change of nutrients or complex substances into simpler compounds, accompanied by a release of energy.

Catalyst: a substance that modifies, especially increases, the rate of chemical reaction without being consumed or changed in the process.

Chelation: a process by which mineral substances are changed into easily digestible form.

Chronic: a long duration; continuing; constant.

Coenzyme: the major portion, though nonprotein, part of an enzyme; usually a B vitamin.

Collagen: the primary organic constituent of bone, cartilage, and connective tissue (becomes gelatin through boiling).

Congenital: condition existing at birth, not hereditary.

Dehydration: a condition resulting from an excessive loss of water from the body.

Dermatitis: an inflammation of the skin; a rash.

Desiccated: dried; preserved by removing moisture.

Dicalcium phosphate: a filler used in pills, which is derived from purified mineral rocks and is an excellent source of calcium and phosphorus.

Diluents: fillers; inert material added to tablets to increase their bulk in order to make them a practical size for compression.

Diuretic: tending to increase the flow of urine from the body.

DNA: deoxyribonucleic acid; the nucleic acid in chromosomes that is part of the chemical basis for hereditary characteristics.

Endogenous: being produced from within the body.

Enteric coated: a tablet coated so that it dissolves in the intestine, not in the stomach (which is acid).

Enuresis: bed-wetting.

Enzyme: a protein substance found in living cells that brings about chemical changes; necessary for digestion of food.

Excipient: any inert substance used as a dilutant or vehicle for a drug.

Exogenous: being derived or developed from external causes.

FDA: Food and Drug Administration.

Fibrin: an insoluble protein that forms the necessary fibrous network in the coagulation of blood.

Free-radicals: highly reactive chemical fragments that can produce an irritation of artery walls, start the arteriosclerotic process if vitamin E is not present; genrally harmful.

Fructose: a natural sugar occurring in fruits and honey; called fruit sugar; often used as a preservative for foodstuffs and an intravenous nutrient.

Galactosemia: a hereditary disorder in which milk becomes toxic as food.

Glucose: blood sugar; a product of the body's assimilation of carbohydrates and a major source of energy.

Glutamic acid: an amino acid present in all complete proteins; usually manufactured from vegetable protein; used as a salt substitute and a flavor-intensifying agent.

Glutamine: an amino acid that constitutes, with glucose, the major nourishment used by the nervous system.

Gluten: a mixture of two proteins—gliadin and glutenin—present in wheat, rye, oats, and barley.

Glycogen: the body's chief storage carbohydrate, primarily in the liver.

GRAS: Generally Recognized As Safe; a list established by Congress to cover substances added to food.

Hesperidin: part of the C complex.

Holistic treatment: treatment of the whole person.

Homeostasis: the body's physiological equilibrium.

Hormone: a substance formed in endocrine organs and transported by body fluids to activate other specifically receptive organs.

Humectant: a substance that is used to preserve the moisture content of materials.

Hydrochloric acid: a normally acidic part of the body's gastric juice.

Hydrolyzed: put into water-soluble form.

Hydrolyzed protein chelate: water-soluble and chelated for easy assimilation.

Hypervitaminosis: a condition caused by an excessive ingestion of vitamins.

Hypoglycemia: a condition caused by abnormally low blood sugar.

Hypovitaminosis: a deficiency disease owing to an absence of vitamins in the diet.

Ichthyosis: a condition characterized by a scaliness on the outer layer of skin.

Idiopathic: a condition whose causes are not yet known.

Immune: protected against disease.

Insulin: the hormone, secreted by the pancreas, concerned with the metabolism of sugar in the body.

IU: International Units.

Lactating: producing milk.

Laxative: a substance that stimulates evacuation of the bowels.

Linoleic acid: one of the polyunsaturated fats, a constituent of lecithin; known as vitamin F; indispensable for life, and must be obtained from foods.

Lipid: a fat or fatty substance.

Lipofuscin: age pigment in cells.

Lipotropic: preventing abnormal or excessive accumulation of fat in the liver.

Megavitamin therapy: treatment of illness with massive amounts of vitamins.

Metabolize: to undergo change by physical and chemical processes.

Nitrites: used as fixatives in cured meats; can combine with natural stomach and food chemicals to cause dangerous cancer-causing agents called nitrosamines.

Orthomolecular: the right molecule used for the right treatment; doctors who practice preventive medicine and use vitamin therapies are known as orthomolecular physicians.

OSHA: Occupational Safety and Health Administration.

Oxalates: organic chemicals found in certain foods, especially spinach, which can combine with calcium to form calcium oxalate, an insoluble chemical the body cannot use.

PABA: para-aminobenzoic acid; a member of the B complex.

Palmitate: water-solublized vitamin A.

PKU (phenylketonuria): a hereditary disease caused by the lack of an enzyme needed to convert an essential amino acid (phenylalanine) into a form usable by the body; can cause mental retardation unless detected early.

Polyunsaturated fats: highly nonsaturated fats from vegetable sources; tend to lower blood cholesterol.

Predigested protein: protein that has been processed for fast assimilation and can go directly to the bloodstream.

Provitamin: a vitamin precursor; a chemical substance necessary to produce a vitamin.

PUFA: poylunsaturated fatty acid.

RDA: Recommended Dietary Allowances as established by the Food and Nutrition Board, National Academy of Sciences, National Research Council.

RNA: the abbreviation used for ribonucleic acid.

Rose hips: a rich source of vitamin C; the nodule underneath the bud of a rose called a hip, in which the plant produces the vitamin C we extract.

Rutin: a substance extracted from buckwheat; part of the C complex.

Saturated fatty acids: usually solid at room temperature; higher proportions found in foods from animal sources; tend to raise blood cholesterol levels.

Sequestrant: a substance that absorbs ions and prevents changes that would affect flavor, texture, and color of food; used for water softening.

Syncope: brief loss of consciousness; fainting.

Synergistic: the action of two or more substances to produce an effect that neither alone could accomplish.

Synthetic: produced artificially.

Systemic: capable of spreading through the entire body.

Teratological: monstrous or abnormal formations in animals or plants.

Tocopherols: the group of compounds (alpha, beta, delta, epsilon, eta, gamma, and zeta) that make vitamin E; obtained through vacuum distillation of edible vegetable oils.

Toxicity: the quality or condition of being poisonous, harmful, or destructive.

Toxin: an organic poison produced in living or dead organisms.

Triglycerides: fatty substances in the blood.

Unsaturated fatty acids: most often liquid at room temperature; primarily found in vegetable fats.

USAN: United States Adopted Names Council; cosponsored by the American Pharmaceutical Association (APhA), the American Medical Association (AMA), and the United States Pharmacopia (USP) for the specific purpose of coining suitable, acceptable, nonproprietary names in the drug field.

USRDA: United States Recommended Daily Allowances.
Xerosis: a condition of dryness.
Zein: protein from corn.
Zyme: a fermenting substance.

Bibliography and Recommended Reading

The following list is given to show my sincere appreciation for the many nutritionists, scientists, doctors, professors, researchers, and concerned parents whose work in the field of vitamins in general, and children's nutrition in particular, provided the bedrock of my knowledge and proved indispensable in the preparation of this project.

Although many of the books are highly technical and written for professionals in the field, there are others—which I have marked with an asterisk—that I highly recommend to parents, whose interest I hope I've sparked, for further reading in pursuit of healthier, happier children.

*ABRAHAMSON, E. M., AND PEZET, A. W. *Body, Mind and Sugar*. New York: Holt, Rinehart and Winston, 1951.

*ADAMS, RUTH. *The Complete Home Guide to All the Vitamins*. New York: Larchmont Books, 1972.

*———, AND MURRAY, FRANK. *Minerals: Kill or Cure*. New York: Larchmont Books, 1976.

*AGUILAR, NONA. *Totally Natural Beauty*. New York: Rawson Associates Publishers, 1977.

*AIROLA, PAAVO. *Are You Confused?* Phoenix, Ariz.: Health Plus, 1972.

*———. *How to Get Well*. Phoenix, Ariz.: Health Plus, 1975.

*———. *Hypoglycemia, A Better Approach*. Phoenix, Ariz.: Health Plus, 1977.

*ARNOW, L. EARLE. *Food Power: A Doctor's Guide to Commonsense Nutrition*. Chicago: Nelson-Hall, 1972.

*ATKINS, ROBERT C. *Dr. Atkins' Diet Revolution*. New York: David McKay, 1972.

*BAILEY, HUBERT. *Vitamin E: Your Key to a Healthy Heart*. New York: ARC Books, 1964, 1966.

BIERI, JOHN G. "Fat-soluble Vitamins in the Eighth Revision of the Recommended Dietary Allowances." *Journal of the American Dietetic Association* 64 (February 1974).

Blood: The River of Life. American National Red Cross, 1976.

BOGERT, JEAN; BRIGGS, GEORGE M.; AND CALLOWAY, DORIS HOWES. *Nutrition and Physical Fitness*. Philadelphia: W. B. Saunders Company, 1973.

*BORSAAK, HENRY. *Vitamins: What They Are and How They Can Benefit You*. New York: Pyramid Books, 1971.

"Bread: You Can't Judge a Loaf by Its Color." *Consumer Reports* 41 (May 1976).

*BRICKLIN, MARK. *Practical Encyclopedia of Natural Healing*. Emmaus, Pa.: Rodale Press Books, 1976.

BRODY, JANE E. "Cancer-blocking Agents Found in Foods." *The New York Times* (March 6, 1979).

*BURACK, RICHARD. *The New Handbook of Prescription Drugs*. New York: Ballantine, 1967, 1970.

*———, WITH FOX, FRED J. *New Handbook of Prescription Drugs*. New York: Pantheon Books, 1967.

BURTON, BENJAMIN. *Human Nutrition*. 3rd ed. New York: McGraw-Hill, 1976.

"Buying Beef." *Consumer Reports* 39 (September 1974).

CHANEY, MARGARET S., AND ROSS, MARGARET L. *Nutrition*. Boston: Houghton-Mifflin, 1971.

*CLARK, LINDA. *The Best of Linda Clark*. New Canaan, Conn.: Keats Publishing Co., 1976.

*———. *Know Your Nutrition*. New Canaan, Conn.: Keats Publishing Co., 1973.

*———. *Secrets of Health and Beauty*. New York: Jove Publications, 1977.

*Consumer Reports, Editors of. *The Medicine Show*. Mount Vernon, N.Y.: Consumers Union, 1961.

COOPER, L. F.; MITCHELL, H. S.; and others. *Nutrition in Health and Disease*. New York: Lippincott, 1963.

*CRAWFORD, F. M., ed. *American Home All-Purpose Cookbook*. New York: M. Evans and Co., 1972.

*CROOK, WILLIAM G. *Your Child and Allergy*. Jackson, Tenn.: Professional Books, 1977.

Cumulative Index for Journal of Applied Nutrition. La Habra,

Calif.: International College of Applied Nutrition, 1947–76, 1976.

Current Practices in Infant Feeding. Fremont, Mich.: Gerber Products Company, 1980.

*DAVIS, ADELLE. *Let's Eat Right to Keep Fit*. New York: Harcourt, Brace and World, 1954.

*———. *Let's Have Healthy Children*. 2nd ed. New York: Harcourt, Brace and World, 1959.

*———. *Let's Get Well*. New York: Harcourt, Brace and World, 1965.

*DEUTSCH, RONALD M. *The Family Guide to Better Food and Better Health*. Des Moines, Iowa: Meredith Corporation, 1971.

*DUFTY, WILLIAM. *Sugar Blues*. Radnor, Pa.: Chilton Book Co., 1975.

*EBON, MARTIN. *Which Vitamins Do You Need?* New York: Bantam Books, 1974.

"Fast-Food Chains." *Consumer Reports* 44 (September 1979).

FLYNN, MARGARET A. "The Cholesterol Controversy." *Journal of the American Pharmacy* NS18 (May 1978).

"Food Facts Talk Back." *Journal of the American Dietetic Association* (1977).

*FRANK, BENJAMIN S. *No-Aging Diet*. New York: Dial, 1976.

*FREDERICKS, CARLTON. *Eating Right for You*. New York: Grosset and Dunlap, 1972.

*———. *Psycho-Nutrients*. New York: Grosset and Dunlap, 1976.

*GOMEZ, JOAN, AND GERCH, MARVIN J. *Dictionary of Symptoms*. New York: Stein and Day, 1968.

GOODHART, ROBERT S., AND SHILLS, MAURICE E. *Modern Nutrition in Health and Disease*. 5th ed. Philadelphia: Lea and Febiger, 1973.

*GOODWIN, MARY T., AND POLLEN, GERRY. *Creative Food Experiences for Children*. Washington, D.C.: Center for Science in the Public Interest, 1974.

*GRAEDON, JOE. *The People's Pharmacy*. New York: St. Martin's Press, 1976.

A Guide to Planning Meals for Babies with Special Needs. Ft. Washington, Pa.: The Beech-Nut Company, Form #79-13, May 1979.

Guidelines for the Eradication of Iron-Deficiency Anemia. New York: International Nutritional Anemia Consultative Group (INACG), 1976.

Guidelines for the Eradication of Vitamin-A Deficiency and Xerophthalmia. New York: International Vitamin-A Consultative Group (IVACG), 1976.

HARPER, ALFRED E. "Recommended Dietary Allowances: Are They What We Think They Are?" *Journal of the American Dietetic Association* 64 (February 1974).

*HAUSER, GAYLORD. *Treasury of Secrets: A Passport to a New Way of Life.* New York: Farrar, Straus, 1951, 1952, 1955, 1961.

*HESLIN, JO-ANN; NATOW, ANNETTE B.; AND RAVEN, BARBARA. *No-Nonsense Nutrition for Your Baby's First Year.* Boston: CBI Publishing Co., 1978.

HOLVEY, DAVID, ed. *The Merck Manual.* 12th ed. Rahway, N. J.: Merck and Co., 1972.

"Hot Dogs." *Consumer Reports* 45 (May 1980).

"How Nutritious Are Fast-Food Meals?" *Consumer Reports* 40 (May 1975).

HOWE, PHYLLIS S. *Basic Nutrition in Health and Disease.* 6th ed. Philadelphia: W.B. Saunders Co., 1976.

*HUNTER, B. T. *The Natural Foods Primer.* New York: Simon and Schuster, 1972.

Index of Nutrition Education Materials. Washington, D.C.: Nutrition Foundation, 1977.

Ingredients: Gerber Baby Foods. Fremont, Mich.: Gerber Food Co., August 1980.

"Is Breast-Feeding Best for Babies?" *Consumer Reports* 42 (March 1977).

JACOBSON, MICHAEL, AND WILSON, WENDY. *Food Scorecard.* Washington, D.C.: Center for Science in the Public Interest, 1974; rev. 1980 by Jan Zimmerman.

Journal of Applied Nutrition. International College of Applied Nutrition, La Habra, Calif., 1974–76.

*KARELITZ, SAMUEL. *When Your Child Is Ill.* New York: Random House, 1969.

KATZ, MARCELLA. *Vitamins, Food, and Your Health.* Public Affairs Committee, 1971. 1975.

*KORDEL, L. *Health Through Nutrition.* New York: Mac-Fadden-Bartell, 1971.

KRAUS, BARBARA. *The Dictionary of Calories and Carbohydrates*. New York: Grosset and Dunlap, 1974.

LARSEN, GENA. *Better Food for Better Babies and Their Families*. New Canaan, Conn.: Keats Publishing, 1972.

*LINDE, SHIRLEY. *The Whole Health Catalog*. New York: Rawson Associates Publishers, 1977.

*LUCAS, RICHARD. *Nature's Medicines*. New York: Prentice-Hall, 1966.

*MARTIN, CLEMENT G. *Low Blood Sugar: The Hidden Menace of Hypoglycemia*. New York: Arco Publishing Co., 1976.

*MARTIN, MARVIN. *The Great Vitamin Mystery*. Rosemont, Ill.: National Dairy Council, 1978.

MASON, DAVID, AND DYLLER, FRAN. *Pharmaceutical Dictionary and Reference for Prescription Drugs*. New York: Playboy Paperbacks, 1980.

*MAYER, JEAN. *A Diet for Living*. New York: David McKay, 1975.

MITCHELL, HELEN S. "Recommended Dietary Allowances Up to Date." *Journal of the American Dietetic Association* 64 (February 1974).

National Health Federation Bulletin (November 1978).

National Research Council. *Toxicants Occurring Naturally in Foods*. 2nd ed. Washington, D.C.: National Academy of Sciences, 1973.

National Research Council. *Recommended Dietary Allowances*. 8th ed., revised. Washington, D.C.: National Academy of Sciences, 1974.

*NEWBOLD, H. L. *Dr. Newbold's Revolutionary New Discovery about Weight Loss*. New York: Rawson Associates Publishers, 1977.

*————. *Mega-Nutrients for Your Nerves*. New York: Peter H. Wyden, Publisher, 1978.

*NULL, GARY AND STEVE. *The Complete Book of Nutrition*. New York: Dell, 1972.

**Nutrition Almanac*. Nutrition Search, Inc. New York: McGraw-Hill, 1973.

Nutrition and Intellectual Growth in Children. Washington, D.C.: Association for Childhood Education International, 1968–69.

Nutrition—Applied Personally. La Habra, Calif.: International College of Applied Nutrition, 1978.

Nutrition Information Resources for the Whole Family. Washington, D.C.: National Nutrition Education Clearing House, 1978.

Nutrition Labeling: How It Can Work for You. Washington, D.C.: National Nutrition Consortium, American Dietetic Association, 1975.

Nutrition Source Book. Rosemont, Ill.: National Dairy Council, 1978.

*PASSWATER, RICHARD A. *Supernutrition*. New York: Dial, 1975.

*PAULING, LINUS. *Vitamin C and the Common Cold*. New York: Bantam Books, 1971.

PILTZ, ALBERT. *How Your Body Uses Food*. Rosemont, Ill.: National Dairy Council, 1960, 1977.

Planning Meals for the Allergic Infant. Pittsburgh: H. J. Heinz Co., 1980.

*POMERANZ, VIRGINIA E., AND SCHULTZ, DODI. *The Mothers' and Fathers' Medical Encyclopedia*. Boston: Little, Brown, 1977.

"Present Knowledge in Nutrition." *Nutrition Reviews*. Nutrition Foundation, Inc., 1976.

*RODALE, J. I. *The Complete Book of Minerals for Health*. 4th ed. Emmaus, Pa.: Rodale Press Books, 1976.

*———. *The Encyclopedia of Common Diseases*. Emmaus, Pa.: Rodale Press Books, 1976.

*ROSENBERG, HAROLD, AND FELDZMAN, A. N. *Doctor's Book of Vitamin Therapy: Megavitamins for Health*. New York: Putnam's, 1974.

*RUBINSTEIN, MORTON K. *A Doctor's Guide to Non-Prescription Drugs*. New York: New American Library, 1977.

*SCHARLATT, ELISABETH, ed. *Kids: Day in and Day out—A Parents' Manual*. New York: Simon & Schuster, 1979.

*———. *Improving Your Child's Behavior Chemistry*. New York: Simon & Schuster, 1976.

*SMITH, LENDON. *Feed Your Kids Right*. New York: McGraw-Hill, 1979.

*SPOCK, BENJAMIN. *Baby and Child Care*. New York: Simon & Schuster, 1976.

"Too Much Sugar." *Consumer Reports* 43 (March 1978).

Tots at the Table: A Food Guide for Use by Parents with Children from 1 to 5 Years. Chicago: National Livestock and Meat Board, 1979.

UNDERWOOD, ERIC J. *Trace Elements in Human and Animal Nutrition*. 4th ed. New York: Academic Press, 1977.

United Nations. Food and Agriculture Organization. *Calorie Requirements*, 1957, 1972.

U.S. Department of Agriculture. *Amino Acid Content of Food* by M. L. Orr and B.K. Watt, 1957; rev. 1968.

U.S. Department of Agriculture. Consumer and Food Economics Institute, Agricultural Research Service. *Composition of Foods: Raw, Processed, Prepared* by Bernice K. Watt and Annabel L. Merrill, 1975.

U.S. Department of Agriculture. *Energy Value of Foods: Basis and Derivation* by Annabel L. Merrill and Bernice K. Watt, 1973.

U.S. Department of Agriculture. *Nutritive Value of American Foods* by Catherine F. Adams, 1975.

U.S. Department of Health, Education and Welfare. *Ten-State Nutrition Survey*. Washington, D.C.: U.S. Government Printing Office, 1968–70.

U.S. Department of Health, Education and Welfare. *Consumer Health Education: A Directory*, 1975.

"The U.S. Food and Drug Administration: On Food and Drugs." *Consumer Reports* 38 (March 1973).

U.S. President's Council on Physical Fitness and Sports. *Exercise and Weight Control* by Robert E. Johnson. Urbana, Ill.: University of Illinois Press, 1967.

U.S. Senate. Select Committee on Nutrition and Human Needs. *National Nutrition Policy: Nutrition and the Consumer II*. Washington, D.C.: U.S. Government Printing Office, 1974.

U.S. Senate. Select Committee on Nutrition and Human Needs. *Diet and Killer Diseases with Press Reaction and Additional Information*. Washington, D.C.: U.S. Government Printing Office, 1977.

"Vitamin-Mineral Safety, Toxicity and Misuse." *Journal of the American Dietetic Association* (1978).

*WADE, CARLSON. *Magic Minerals*. West Nyack, N.Y.: Parker Publishing Co., 1967.

*————. *Miracle Protein*. West Nyack, N.Y.: Parker Publishing Co., 1975.

"Which Cereal for Breakfast?" *Consumer Reports* 46 (February 1981).

"Which Cereals Are Most Nutritious?" *Consumer Reports* 40 (February 1975).

WILLIAMS, ROGER J. *Nutrition Against Disease*. New York: Pitman Publishers, 1971.

*WINTER, RUTH. *A Consumers' Dictionary of Food Additives*. New York: Crown, 1978.

"Yogurt." *Consumer Reports* 43 (January 1978).

*YUDKIN, JOHN. *Sweet and Dangerous*. New York: Peter H. Wyden, 1972.

INDEX

ABOUT THE AUTHOR

EARL MINDELL is a member of the American Nutrition Society, the National Health Federation, the American Pharmaceutical Association (he has been a pharmacist for over fifteen years), a charter member of the American Academy of the General Practice of Pharmacy, and an associate member of the International College of Applied Nutrition. He and his wife and two children live in Beverly Hills, California.